# *the truth about* homosexuality

## bruce smith jr.

# CONTENTS

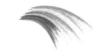

# ACKNOWLEDGEMENTS

To God above all else, for loving and blessing me without measure. To my father, Bruce Smith Sr., for giving me the platform to speak on this subject and inspiring me to write this book. To my mother, Juana Smith, for your consistent support, candor, and excellent recommendations. To my brother, Austin Smith, for your advice and encouragement from the beginning. Thanks for telling me to take a leap of faith. To my cousin, Angela Wood, for pushing me, supporting me, and bridging the gap between author and publisher. To Sylvia Burleigh, for going above and beyond in fighting alongside me to get this book published. To Jennifer Kasper, for guiding me across the finish line. You were each invaluable in this process. I love you all and thank God for you.

# INTRODUCTION

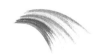

W hat would you say if one of your loved ones "came out" to you as a "homosexual"? How would you council a "homosexual" who asked you for spiritual guidance? What is your response when asked if you're for or against "gay marriage" and why? How do you reconcile what the Bible says about homosexuality with your friends and loved ones who identify as "homosexual"? These are huge questions that can be overwhelming, especially if you're unprepared to answer them. Yet, as Christians we should not only be able to easily answer these questions; all of our answers should be consistent. Unfortunately that is not the case. Many dismiss homosexuality as a topic of unimportance. Others recognize that answering such questions can easily lead to offending people who retaliate with words such as "homophobic," "hateful," "intolerant," and "bigoted." They don't want to be attacked like that so they choose to avoid the issue entirely. While it's certainly easier to keep quiet, is dismissal and avoidance the best response to such an increasingly relevant issue? Not quite.

Homosexuality is a topic that concerns all of humanity, and is addressed repeatedly in the Bible, thus it is too important to ignore or avoid. Further, odds are if you're not struggling with homosexuality yourself, then you know someone who is even if you're unaware of it. If Jesus communicated the truth with love and respect on even the most controversial subjects, Christians are obligated to do likewise. We cannot withhold the truth for fear of persecution. Persecution will come to us anyway. More importantly, "God has not given us a spirit of fear, but of power and of love and of a sound mind" (2 Timothy 1:7, NKJV). I believe it is healthy and helpful to discuss homosexuality provided the discussion is approached from the best standpoint, it is grounded in truth, and everyone remains respectful even while disagreeing.

Unfortunately, when it comes to addressing homosexuality many either don't know the facts, or they are torn between the facts and how they feel. This leaves them in a position where they don't quite know what to think, which only adds to the confusion surrounding the issue. Legitimate questions and struggles persist on all sides, and the line between fact and fiction has become such a blur that the truth has been largely obscured. Both proponents and opponents of homosexuality have often formed an opinion first, planted their feet firmly on that opinion, and insist they're right and all opposing positions are wrong. Of course, everyone can't be right. So how do we determine who is right and who is wrong? What is the resolution? The resolution is truth. Truth has the unique power to change lives and save souls. It is through the truth that questions can be answered correctly, solutions can be discovered, and life struggles can be conquered. The good news is everyone can know the truth about homosexuality if they're open to receiving that truth. So even if you've already formed an opinion on this polarizing topic, as we examine the facts, I challenge you to be open-minded and to accept whatever truth the facts lead to. You may discover what you are convinced is true is not true after all.

### Who Am I to Talk About Homosexuality?
I have never experienced same-sex attraction (SSA), and I do not identify myself as "gay." Therefore, I cannot possibly

speak on homosexuality from a personal experience with homosexuality. So what qualifies me to speak on homosexuality with any authority whatsoever? Firstly, I would submit to you my personal passion for sexual morality. I am a Christian and at a young age I made a vow to remain sexually pure. I am currently in my late thirties and I remain a single, celibate virgin and I will maintain that status until marriage, death, or the return of Christ—whichever comes first. I've never masturbated before and I never will. I don't even watch sexually explicit scenes on TV shows or movies despite my intense attraction to women. I am thoroughly and enduringly dedicated to honoring God with my body by remaining sexually pure. How is this possible? I value God's commandments more than I value pleasure, which sadly is a rarity in today's sex-driven society. It's quite easy for someone who's married and can have sex to their heart's content to tell others it's not right for them to have sex. Though what they're saying might be true, it's often difficult for the listener to accept because the speaker isn't actually living that reality. In my case, I'm living that reality every day and can speak on sexual purity from personal experience. "I've been there and done that," is a powerful position in itself, but "I *am* there and I'm *doing* that," is a far more powerful position.

Secondly, I would submit my passion for the truth. One of the primary reasons homosexuality is such a controversial topic is because the truth is muddled. Homosexuality is riddled with polarizing ideas and concepts, so those who take up positions on opposing sides both believe they are standing on the truth. Obviously, this cannot be so because if everyone stood on the truth, there would be no confusion or controversy. It takes a passion and dedication to the truth to expose what is false and combat confusion with clarity to expose the actual truth. This is what I aim to do here. I believe personal experience plus truth equals a powerful message that can inspire positive change. In order to speak the truth one must first know the truth. So before I could broach this topic with any credibility, it was imperative to do thorough research and come to a clear understanding for myself. I began researching the many facets of homosexuality several years ago. In addition to examining credible resources about homosexuality, I've gone straight to the source as often as possible to gain a comprehensive understanding: I've personally interacted with "ex-gays", those currently struggling with homosexuality, as well as "out and proud homosexuals" and "bisexuals." In addition, I've studied the personal accounts of a host of individuals who fall into these categories. It was through this experience I discovered the truth about homosexuality. This book is a culmination of my research, personal experience, and the resulting logical conclusions.

Thirdly, I have a deep passion for people. Every true Christian has a passion and love for people and a heart for helping those in need. This requires listening, building relationships, and sharing the truth in love as led by the Holy Spirit. My passion for helping people (in this case those who struggle with and those who promote homosexuality) has led to innumerable discussions and debates on the topic. I've also been fortunate to have multiple speaking engagements: twice I was invited to speak at a large purity conference in Raleigh, North Carolina. A secular San Francisco radio station interviewed me about sexual purity. I also continue to speak at churches, talk to youth groups, and privately counsel individuals from all over the world who are struggling with sexual purity.

Part of this passion for people includes being able to relate to their struggles. Again, while I cannot fully relate to those who struggle with homosexuality, there are some aspects of their experience that I can indeed relate to. It is no secret that those who experience SSA and identify as "gay" often have troubled pasts. In listening to their stories, you will most likely hear a common theme: they'll tell you the difficulties they've had fitting in; they'll explain how they felt different from everyone else, and how they were ostracized, bullied, and teased as a result. They'll tell you how they continued to wrestle with questions such as: "Is there something wrong with me?" and "Would the world be better off without me?" They will tell you about a past dedicated to the pursuit of love and acceptance, which resulted in rejection and disappointment instead. Finally they will describe how powerful those negative experiences were and how the impact of those negative experiences continues to plague them to this day.

If I were to tell you my life story you would hear the exact same theme. Although the cause of my negative experiences is not related to homosexuality, the results are no less significant. I've lived through these negative experiences and continue to deal with residual effects. From fourth grade through high school, I was laughed at, bullied, and ridiculed about everything from the way I laughed, to the way I dressed, to the way I ran, to what I packed for lunch. I was called every name in the book, including "gay." This was baffling to me because I was always chasing girls at school, even though I was rejected by *every single one* of them. I even tried to alter my personality in an effort to win the affection of one of those girls, but that too failed.

So yes I've asked myself that horrible question: "Is there something wrong with me?" Yes, I've wondered how the world would be without me in it. I know what all of that is like. The challenges continue. In the radio interview I mentioned, the show's three DJs discussed how waiting until marriage to have sex is virtually taboo in today's liberal culture. They insinuated adult virgins didn't exist and I was pleased to provide a counterargument. The DJs pulled no punches with their direct questions. They asked me how often I masturbated, and when I finally convinced them that I don't and never have, they asked me if I was "gay," followed by: "Are you *sure* you're not 'gay?'" When I finally convinced them I wasn't, they asked if I was "asexual." They couldn't fathom the fact that I was a celibate man in my thirties, so they desperately tried to fit me into a box that made sense to them.

I get questioned by guys who think there is something wrong with me for being celibate, and I've been cheated on in virtually every relationship I've been in because I was not willing to compromise in the area of sex. Most recently, a fellow high school alumnus (a rather cruel atheist and staunch supporter of homosexuality) accused me of being a "deranged and confused self-hating 'homosexual' who tries to hide his identity by becoming a minister." An entire life filled with experiences like these has made me intimately familiar with being the weird one who doesn't fit in. I know exactly how it is to feel an inch tall, to be the butt of jokes, to be made fun of for things I can't help, to be constantly rejected, ridiculed, and questioned. I know how it feels to have nobody to talk to who truly understands because there's nobody around who shares my experience. So while I'm unqualified to provide that experience-based support for those I talk to who are currently struggling with homosexuality, I'm not alien to everything they've endured. This is significant because if I was able to prevent my negative experiences from crushing me and leading me to depression and ultimately suicide, then there is hope for those who are headed in that direction.

I believe my life experience coupled with my passion for sexual morality, truth, and people create a rather unique and effective platform from which to address the issue of homosexuality with authority. Because I personally fight daily for sexually purity in my own life, I am abundantly familiar with the struggles, thoughts, and temptations that come with intense sexual attraction, which is a core component of homosexuality.

With that established, I must make several things perfectly clear before we continue:

- I do *not* hate "homosexuals." I love "homosexuals," which is why I've written this book.
- I recognize not everyone believes what I believe, and while I think it's wrong to force my beliefs on anyone, I do believe it is fruitful to present the truth for consideration.
- I find it deplorable to be disrespectful or cruel to anyone, regardless if they agree with my position or not. It is okay for people to respectfully disagree.
- In preparation for writing this book, I could not afford to make assumptions. This means I had to be open to listening, and I had to focus on facts instead of opinions in order to reach accurate conclusions about homosexuality.

## Sincere Apology

I would like to begin by issuing a sincere apology to anyone who identifies as a "homosexual" who was chastised, made fun of, or attacked (verbally or physically) by anyone who claims to be a Christian. Such behavior is unacceptable, it is totally contrary to the tenets of Christianity, and is appalling to true Christians. Please understand not everyone who claims to be a Christian is truly a Christian. So to those who have suffered ill treatment under the guise of Christianity, I first offer you a sincere apology from a *true Christian*. Secondly, if you determined all Christians were evil or cruel as a result of that unfortunate experience, I would ask that you give me a chance to show you what true Christianity is all about.

## What to Expect

I know a man who is uncomfortable with taking a firm position for or against homosexuality, so he loves to read opinion-based books about homosexuality. He recommended a book to me and said, "It doesn't really answer any questions; it's more of an informative book about homosexuality." He was absolutely right. There is an abundance of difficult questions surrounding homosexuality, and that book didn't answer any of them. As a result, it was an extremely frustrating read. It is not my intention to frustrate you in this manner by only scratching the surface of homosexuality. We're not going to dance around the topic; we're going to put homosexuality under a microscope and lay bare what we observe.

Please note that this is not a "doom and gloom" type of book. It's not a judgmental, finger pointing, "sending people to hell" kind of book. Here you will find the facts and answers to critical questions that will assist you in dealing with the difficult issue of homosexuality. This information is dedicated to helping people from a place of love, respect, compassion, and truth. I must also stress this book is not based on my opinions, because my opinions do not matter: *only the facts matter*. This principle is evident in opinion versus opinion arguments, which unfortunately appear to be far more common than fact-based arguments. Opinion versus opinion arguments are futile because the objective of each side is not to ascertain the truth, but to prove their opinion is "right" and the opposing opinions are "wrong." As a result, these arguments are rarely settled because in the end both sides walk away with the same preconceived notion they started with. On the contrary, arguments based on facts are the most powerful because they are grounded on evidence and proof. For example, it would not be difficult to argue: "Excessive alcohol consumption can result in alcohol poisoning," because this argument is factual, and evidence can be easily provided to prove that it is true. The person who replies by saying, "No it can't," is not stating a fact, but their opinion. Regardless of their reasoning, adamantly arguing an opinion doesn't make that opinion a fact, nor does it make the fact countering that opinion in anyway untrue. One of the most impactful lessons I've learned is this:

*The truth doesn't stop being the truth simply because we disagree with it, disbelieve it, or dislike it. The truth remains the truth regardless of our feelings and opinions.*

I challenge you to consider this carefully and grasp how critical this principle is to growing and learning. Just as my opinions are absolutely irrelevant on the matter of homosexuality, yours are as well. The goal here is not to voice our opinions, but to uncover the truth. When we know the truth, we will be able to accurately answer the critical questions about homosexuality, which will enlighten us, help us, and equip us to enlighten and help others as well.

**Terminology**
To eliminate confusion going forward, I need to lay some groundwork and be extremely clear on what I mean when I use certain words.

> *HOMOSEXUALITY:* erotic behavior with members of the same gender.
> *"HOMOSEXUAL"/"GAY"/ "LESBIAN":* an individual who finds himself or herself sexually attracted to members of the same gender.
> *PRACTICING "HOMOSEXUAL":* an individual whose lifestyle involves the willful engagement in erotic behavior with members of the same gender.
> *"LGBT" ACTIVIST:* "lesbian", "gay", "bisexual", "transgender" individuals, and advocates who vigorously promote and defend homosexuality and "gay rights."
> *"EX-GAY":* an individual who has renounced the homosexual lifestyle and identity.

***ADVOCATE:*** an individual who is not a "homosexual" but passionately promotes and defends homosexuality.
***SSA:*** same-sex attraction.
***OSA:*** opposite-sex attraction.

Now notice we've already uncovered a great deal simply by defining these terms. First notice homosexuality is not limited to "homosexuals." There are individuals who aren't "gay" that engage in homosexuality as well. This may fall into the category of "experimentation" or "exploring one's sexuality," or even be a product of environment such as prisoners who seek sexual gratification from one another. By today's standards, these individuals aren't necessarily classified as "homosexuals," however, this behavior still qualifies as homosexuality. There are actually "straight" men who molest male children. In doing so these pedophiles are also indulging in homosexuality. This is an important distinction because we now see homosexuality is not a subject that only affects one group of people. It has a much wider scope than many people realize.

Secondly, notice there is a difference between a "homosexual" and a practicing "homosexual." A man might identify himself as "gay", but never actually express that identity in actions. In other words, he might have discovered he is attracted to other men but never physically engages in erotic activity with other men. A practicing "homosexual," on the other hand, is someone who is actively engaged in erotic activity with same-sex partners. Keep these important distinctions in mind as we continue.

**Lessons from Personal Experience**
I've learned a great deal from interacting with "homosexuals" and advocates over the years. While some people feel warranted in heaping hatred and cruelty upon "homosexuals"

in some twisted effort to reform them, I've never taken that approach because that is *totally* contrary to Christianity. Though I may not understand or approve of what someone does, that doesn't give me the right to mistreat or disrespect that person, especially knowing plenty of people don't understand or approve of what I do. I certainly don't think that gives them the right to mistreat or disrespect me. I wrongfully assumed as a result of my peaceful and respectful position that I would be spared the fury and negative reactions incited by those who are indeed hateful. I quickly learned *anyone* who is opposed to homosexuality is fair game. This was made abundantly clear to me through social media. Although the whole purpose of social media is free expression, there are quite a few advocates who believe free expression isn't entirely free, and have therefore appointed themselves "censorship police." In their minds it is acceptable for anyone to publicly express their support of homosexuality, but it is strictly forbidden to publicly express nonsupport of homosexuality. Anyone who violates unwritten laws like this one will often suffer the consequences of their wrath.

I found this to be the case whenever I even broached the topic of homosexuality online, despite the fact that I never did so in a hateful fashion. In fact, the first time I addressed the issue was in response to a friend of mine I've known for over twenty years. She was a "lesbian" at the time who was admittedly avoiding God and was frustrated her life was in shambles. I replied to her candid post and suggested instead of continuing down the same path that hadn't yielded any positive results all those years, to finally give God a chance and see what happens. She responded by thanking me for always being there for her, always being willing to tell her the truth, and never judging her. Her advocate friends, on the other hand, went ballistic as though I had done something horrible. They proceeded to berate me with insults and all sorts of foul names even though I had done nothing wrong.

The second time I broached the topic of homosexuality online was also in response to a friend's post. It was an extremely respectful message explaining that although she didn't agree with homosexuality, she felt she had the right to express her views just as those who agree with homosexuality have a right to express theirs. She made it clear that expressing one's views doesn't have to be a negative thing if it is done in a positive way. I agreed with my friend, so I simply shared her post. This proved to be equivalent to lighting the fuse of a dynamite stick. Sharing her message spawned a lengthy and vigorous debate from people who took great offense to it. Shockingly, those who were most offended and lashed out against me the fiercest were professing Christians.

The post that came two years later was one of my own. I spent more than half an hour making sure there was nothing offensive in my message. In fact, the post was entirely positive, and yet it didn't matter. Had I actually written a hateful message, I would have received the same harsh reaction from my friends who were clearly both angered and offended. Even people who have never "liked" or commented on anything I've ever posted immediately unleashed their fury. Strong opposition from my own friends followed as though I'd committed some serious crime. Oddly, no one could tell me what I said that was so offensive. No one would admit it, but the truth was they were offended because I had the audacity to post a message that was not in favor of homosexuality.

What I found most interesting was none of my "gay" friends had any issue with what I posted. One of them not only "liked" the post but also commented she agreed. Later a friend of mine invited me to talk to his "lesbian" roommate about my post (a young lady I'd never met), and she too agreed with what I said. So there was clearly a palpable disconnect between the "homosexuals" I know and the advocates I know. I've *never* been branded as hateful, intolerant, or "homophobic" by any "homosexuals" I know, but I have been repeatedly ridiculed in such fashion by advocates. I found this contrast both perplexing and disturbing. It makes absolutely no sense for advocates to loudly proclaim "hate" is wrong, but then respond to those opposed to homosexuality with hatred. Experiences such as these have taught me some valuable lessons:

**1. Many people have strong *feelings* and *opinions* on homosexuality.**
Everyone has feelings and opinions, and everyone has a right to express their feelings and opinions. The trouble comes when individuals attempt to force their opposition to remain silent, devalue their position, or attempt to force them to alter their position. Unfortunately, in this battle of "My feelings and opinions are right and yours are wrong," facts and reason fall by the wayside.

**2. Many advocates are easily offended and quick to attack those who oppose homosexuality.**
As I expected my advocate friends to know me well enough to recognize I'm not a hateful person, I realized I know them well enough to recognize they aren't hateful people either. So what caused such volatile reactions from them? Why is it easy to have a respectful conversation or debate about homosexuality with some people but not others? After a great deal of time and thought, I discovered it was most often the result of at least one of the following reasons: a personal bias, an anti-Christian worldview, or a misunderstanding of morality.

Those with a personal bias are so close to the issue that it's difficult for them to be objective. They take any opposition to homosexuality personally because to them it is a highly personal matter. They've adopted a "bullies vs. victims" mentality and often draw a direct link from comments made about homosexuality to a specific "homosexual" or group of "homosexuals." I'll give you an example. Let's say Denise tells her friend Tracy, "I personally disapprove of homosexuality." Tracy's favorite cousin Steve happens to be a practicing "homosexual", and so what Tracy actually hears Denise say is, "I personally disapprove of your favorite cousin Steve." So in Tracy's mind, Denise is immediately branded a bully, and her cousin Steve is instantly the victim. This of course sparks negative emotions, which in turn causes Tracy to respond harshly toward Denise, even though Denise is Tracy's friend and she had no ill intent in expressing her view on homosexuality.

Those with an anti-Christian worldview have often been tormented by someone who wasn't truly a Christian and behaved in an abhorrent manner. It is possible that they were also shunned by a true Christian who simply failed to understand how to be loving and respectful while holding to the truth of God's word. Others simply know the Bible forbids homosexuality and they disagree. So they rationalize their feelings by claiming the Bible is false (for any variety of reasons) and determine Christianity must therefore be false as well. The irony is both true Christians and advocates share something in common: they want to *help* "homosexuals," not *harm* them. The difference is in the methodology. The advocate's idea of helping "homosexuals" is to leave them alone and allow them to do whatever they wish under the guise of love and tolerance. The Christian idea of helping "homosexuals" is to tell them the truth; to save them from a dangerous and immoral lifestyle in a loving and respectful way to ensure they not only have an abundant life here on earth, but they secure their eternal place in heaven as well.

Those with a misunderstanding of morality believe they have the power to establish what is good and evil, and what is right and wrong, when in fact they are simply asserting their *opinion* of what is good and evil, and what is right and wrong, as though it is factual. In other words, if one person says homosexuality is morally wrong, and another person says it is morally right, homosexuality can't be both morally wrong and morally right. It's either one or the other, which means one person is actually correct, and the other person is incorrect. Obviously, the moral status of an issue is not determined by someone's opinion or even a group of opinions. Morality (as we will learn later) can only be established by a perfect moral agent, which none of us are. Nevertheless, for those who misunderstand morality, anyone who disagrees with their claim that there's nothing wrong with homosexuality are dismissed as being "wrong."

**3. Many people base their view of homosexuality on a small fraction of the "homosexual" community instead of homosexuality in its entirety.**
The common advocate mentality is, "All the 'homosexuals' I know are good, funny, loving people, and so there's nothing wrong with homosexuality." This is like looking through a window into a room of a tall building and basing your opinion of the entire building on the small fraction that you see. You obviously couldn't accurately assess the condition of the entire building based on such a limited perspective. Likewise, there is a lot more to homosexuality than what many people are aware of. Homosexuality is a worldwide phenomenon that directly or indirectly affects all of us. The climate of homosexuality cannot be judged by the personal relationships we have with "homosexuals" coupled with what we see on TV and in the movies. Mainstream media purposely paints homosexuality in a positive light by showing "homosexuals" as either happy, loving, hilarious, peaceful people, or hopeless victims who suffer constant verbal or physical abuse to inspire tolerance through sympathy. If these extremes were an accurate depiction of homosexuality as a whole, advocates would be warranted in their eagerness to label "homosexuals" as victims and every opposer of homosexuality as

a bully, but this is not at all an accurate depiction. There are far more facets to homosexuality that most people remain oblivious to because it falls outside of their experience. I've personally witnessed what goes on in the dark basement of a "gay" club (long story), I've seen the systematic deterioration of those caught in the "homosexual" lifestyle, I've researched the long list of negative physical and mental effects that result from homosexuality, I've heard the sobering tales of "ex-gays" who confessed what goes on behind closed doors in the "homosexual" community, and it is *nothing* like what the media portrays or what most people witness from their "homosexual" loved ones.

**4. There is great inconsistency on homosexuality even among Christians.**
There are those who strongly approve of homosexuality, and then there are those who strongly disapprove of homosexuality. Even in Christianity some believe that there is nothing wrong with homosexuality and that "homosexuals" should be free to engage in sexual relationships with whomever they wish. Other Christians believe homosexuality is sinful according to the Bible and should therefore be abstained from in order to honor God. Christians are supposed to be united. So how can members of the body of Christ, who are all supposed to be moving in the same direction, be divided on this issue? Both groups certainly can't be right. So who is right and who is wrong? We will find out soon enough.

# I

# What "LGBT" Activists Don't Want You to Know

T he goal of "LGBT" activists is to convince everyone that homosexuality is a normal, natural, moral, healthy, and fun-filled lifestyle, which should be embraced and encouraged. To accomplish this they continue their long-standing tradition of painting homosexuality in a lovely light, while praising those who accept it, and demonizing those who oppose it. This has been an incredibly successful campaign. A few decades ago homosexuality was widely considered taboo while today it is a global phenomenon. It's trendy; it's what's "in" right now. To come out as a "homosexual" is to be met with applause by the media and secular society for being fun, fashionable, and progressive. This is all a part of "LGBT" activists' design, and the masses are drinking the Kool-Aid by the gallon. It is truly amazing how many people have made up their minds and taken up a firm stance on homosexuality without ever examining the facts, asking any questions, or doing any research. They never paused to ask, "are 'LGBT' activists even telling the truth?" This is a fundamental question because if "LGBT" activists are being honest, and homosexuality is everything they say it is, then everyone, including Christians, should join in the celebration and embrace the lifestyle. If, however, they are not being honest, then homosexuality is not what they say it is, which begs the question: what are they not telling us and why? Could it be that homosexuality is actually an abnormal, unnatural, immoral, unhealthy and danger-filled lifestyle? While "LGBT" activists and homosexuality supporters are convinced this is impossible, what do the facts tell us? After all, one cannot hope to make an informed decision without first examining the facts. Without the facts we will not know the truth. Yet many of those who lack all the pieces to the puzzle insist they have enough to see the full picture when they don't. Our objective is to avoid this. We cannot afford to be ignorant, confused, or deceived when it comes to matters where people's lives and souls are hanging in the balance. So let's shift our focus from proving that our preconceived notions about homosexuality are right, to uncovering the truth. Let's determine we will not be among the ignorant—who don't know the facts, the confused—who don't understand the facts, or the deceived—who don't believe the facts. Let's be among the knowledgeable who know the facts, who have uncovered the truth, and have based our position on that truth. This requires us to shine a searchlight under the rainbow flag and examine what is hiding beneath it. This requires us to uncover the secrets that "LGBT" activists don't want exposed because it would devastate their entire agenda. So what are these little-known facts about homosexuality? What lurks beneath the rainbow banner that most people are unaware of? Let's take a look.

## "LGBT" Activists have a Secret Agenda

The "homosexual" movement operates both overtly and covertly and is making tremendous strides often completely under the radar. It is no secret "LGBT" activists have an agenda. They've publicized it well: to normalize homosexuality and fight for "gay rights" by promoting love, equality, tolerance, etc. It all sounds positive. What is lesser known is the fact that they have a *secret* agenda. The "gay rights" movement is merely a component of the broader campaign called the Sexual Freedom Movement, which is essentially an extension of the Sexual Revolution that began in the sixties. The purpose of the Sexual Freedom Movement is to redefine the nature of all sexual conduct, replacing morality with boundless pleasure to create an entirely new "anything goes" sexual culture. We've already seen the results of this movement in today's increasingly liberal culture that celebrates and promotes nudity, pornography, masturbation, premarital sex, polygamy, polyamory (open sexual relationships), bestiality, incest, pedophilia, and homosexuality. This strategic campaign has been successfully implemented over time, and it continues to redefine every sexual practice that has historically been deemed taboo. This is obviously an immoral and dangerous campaign because devious sexual behavior comes with a host of negative consequences including death. However, "LGBT" activists believe achieving boundless pleasure is worth all the risks.

## Today's "Progressive" Philosophy on Human Sexuality is False

The "gay rights" movement has had tremendous success because of today's progressive-minded culture. The thinking is that in all areas "old is bad and new is good." This means that everything traditional and sacred is now dismissed, and new ideas are embraced with no regard to morality. Restriction is despised, and freedom is praised—sexual freedom in particular. So in order to achieve that freedom, everything that has historically been deemed right and good has been picked apart and painted as wrong and evil, while that which is wrong and evil has been dressed up and presented as right and good. Such is the war that has been waged on morality. So how does this relate to human sexuality? "LGBT" activists have perpetrated this "progressive" philosophy that essentially says:

> *Everyone is a sexual being. Your sexuality is to be fully embraced. Don't be ashamed. Don't fight your sexual urges; give in to them. Explore your body and unlock the mystery of your sexuality. If you don't know what your sexual preference is, experiment until you find out. In discovering your sexual preferences, you've established your sexual orientation, which defines your sexual identity. At that point you know how to live a healthy and fulfilling lifestyle based on your sexual identity.*

In short the message is simply "open yourself to lust and go wherever it takes you." Though this philosophy is dangerous and entirely false, this is the message that the world has widely accepted. This is the message that is being communicated to our children. Further, the results of accepting this philosophy have proven disastrous. Sexually transmitted diseases, infections, unplanned pregnancies, abortions, adultery, divorce, rape, pornography, pedophilia, and bestiality are just a few direct consequences of unbridled lust and the rates in which they occur continue to skyrocket. In the days of old, these practices were abhorred. In godly cultures sex was regarded as a holy and sacred act reserved only for a husband and wife. People had respect for one another, they practiced self-control, abstinence, celibacy, monogamy, and the consequences were blessed marriages, loving families, and healthy individuals. Look at the difference in consequences between that time and this. It's obvious the path to truly healthy and fulfilling sexual lifestyles has nothing to do with lust. This concept that indulging in boundless pleasure is the height of human existence is a fallacy. In fact, quite the opposite is true. Those who have exhausted themselves with pleasure are not left satisfied in the end but broken and depressed. World-renowned theologian Ravi Zacharias put it like this:

> *Some of the loneliest people I have met or read about are those who have had everything and experience little of what we usually consider pain; yet, they too have pain—pain resulting from having indulged and come away empty. The greatest disappointment (and resulting pain) you can feel is when you have just experienced that which you thought would bring you the ultimate in pleasure—and it has let you down. Pleasure without boundaries produces a life without purpose. This is real pain. No death, no tragedy, no atrocity—nothing really matters. Life is sheer hollowness, with no purpose.*[1]

I've seen this myself. The two most promiscuous people I've ever personally known have both had more sexual exploits than they can probably count, and they were both absolutely miserable people. One is a male, the other a female, and neither was able to find satisfaction in their wild and promiscuous sexual encounters. Both turned to alcohol and drugs as a means to ease their depression but nothing worked until they realized the height of life was not found in sexual pleasure like many are led to believe.

## The Terms "Heterosexual" and "Homosexual" Were Invented in an Effort to Normalize Homosexuality

This was a complete shock to me. I still remember learning the difference between a "homosexual" and a "heterosexual" in ninth grade biology class and from that day on I thought these were valid biological terms. They aren't. They were completely made up in the late 1800s. Not by a behavioral scientist, biologist, or geneticist, but by a journalist who was on a mission to repeal sodomy laws. Now why is the invention and global acceptance of these terms significant? Firstly, these terms have no scientific credence of any kind, which immediately disproves many pro-homosexual arguments.

Secondly, this has had a monumental impact on our culture in favor of homosexuality. Instantly a narrative was created that established the idea that there is a sexual dichotomy to humanity (like the two sides of one coin), which suggests equality. In other words, the idea is "heterosexuals" and "homosexuals" are equal even though they are different.

Thirdly, it has distracted everyone from focusing on the moral status of homosexuality. Historically homosexuality (or sodomy) was a behavior that was deemed immoral. Thus to indulge in homosexuality was to commit an immoral act. Today it is commonly held that homosexuality is no longer a behavior, it is an identity that is simply different from the "heterosexual" identity. So a "heterosexual" identity drives heterosexual behavior as a "homosexual" identity drives homosexual behavior. This has created a justification for homosexuality, mainly that it is not something one chooses to do; it is something one does because it is who they are. This set the stage for a number of arguments that have been used to justify homosexuality ever since. One is the assertion that "homosexuals" are born that way, another is the assertion that homosexuality isn't immoral. If the "homosexual" is born that way, then that justifies homosexuality, and if the "homosexual" is an otherwise moral person, how can they be immoral simply for behaving the way they are wired to? This suggests homosexuality isn't immoral in itself; so there is no reason to oppose it any longer. Notice the entire focus has shifted from the *behavior* to the *person*. Suddenly condemning homosexuality has somehow become equivalent to condemning all "homosexuals." It's been made personal and such condemnation is considered hateful because it damages their self-perception and infringes on their human rights. The thinking is: "Heterosexuals" have a right to love, so "homosexuals" do too. So like mistreating a person because he is black is racist, and like mistreating a woman because of her gender is sexist, now opposing homosexuality is considered mistreating "homosexuals," which is "homophobic." "Homosexuals" have been recognized as a class, which was the goal because those who are in a class have rights. This gave rise to the "gay rights" movement, which "LGBT" activists compare to the women's rights, and civil rights movements to gain sympathy and support. How has this affected our culture? Now our top priority is not to maintain a moral lifestyle but to not offend "homosexuals" regardless if their lifestyle is immoral or not. Thus in appeasing "homosexuals" by not challenging homosexuality, one appeases homosexuality, which was the primary objective all along.

So what happens when we reject these invented terms and everything that follows? The remaining sexual categories are simple, like it was in the beginning: sexually moral, and sexually immoral. This is the way God views mankind in regard to sex, and I prefer to view mankind the way God does.

I don't believe people should be identified by their sexuality, which is why I'm not a proponent of using the invented terms "homosexual", "heterosexual", "gay", "lesbian", or "straight." We are humans and our identity is established at birth long before we even develop sexually. Nevertheless, because most people are familiar with these terms and use them, I will continue to use them throughout this book, but always in quotation marks as you have seen.

## There is No Such Thing as "Sexual Orientation"

With the acceptance of the terms "homosexual" and "heterosexual", people began to question the cause of the difference. What causes some people to be "homosexual" and others to be "heterosexual?" Another term that was invented out of thin air served as the answer. Introducing "sexual orientation." Now all of a sudden, everyone has a "sexual orientation" and it's the "sexual orientation" that defines a person's "sexual identity," which in turn determines their sexual behavior. This is both an attempt to separate an individual's actions from the individual, while further establishing the idea of equality between heterosexuality and homosexuality. The thinking goes: like a "heterosexual's" "sexual orientation" points them in one direction, a "homosexual's" "sexual orientation" points them in another direction similar to the way our palate determines our preference in food; it varies from person to person. This concept has also been widely accepted without any questions asked and now virtually everyone believes "sexual orientation" is actually a thing and they have one. Jason Salamone unapologetically illustrated the absurdity of this in his article *21 Questions for the Tolerance Crowd*[2]:

*I understand that "sexual orientation" refers to romantic or sexual preference. So what scientific method is used to show that "sexual orientation" is real? That is, what is the empirical evidence that homosexuality is a uniform attribute across individuals, has its own DNA, that sexual attraction never fluctuates, and homosexuality can easily be measured? Where is "sexual orientation" located? On the liver? The earlobe? The pancreas? If we have a "sexual orientation" why can't doctors identify our "sexual orientation" when we are born? Do I get it at Wal-Mart in a bucket? Can I get prescription shots of it at my local pharmacy? And does proof of the existence of "sexual orientation" mean that the behavior that flows from it, should be affirmed, encouraged? If "sexual orientation" exists, can you please show me a picture of one? If it is invisible, what kind of instrument do you use to measure it? Electricity is measured by voltage meters. Thoughts can be measured with lie detector devices, and with medical equipment. Meteorologists have instruments to measure wind. Where's the MRI and/or CAT scan data for "sexual orientation?" Can you really not see you have placed blind faith into something very abstract and highly ambiguous? Can you really not see that "sexual orientation" is a concept that takes more faith than logic and reason to believe in?*

Sadly the acceptance of this concept has set a dangerous precedent. On the heels of convincing the world that "sexual orientation" actually exists and justifies homosexuality, other sexually deviant groups including pedophiles and the incestuous are now seeking justification by claiming their behaviors are the product of their "sexual orientation" too.

## There is No Such Thing as a "Sexual Identity"

As we've seen, first came the invention of "homosexual" and "heterosexual" and it was supposedly the "sexual orientation" that is the deciding factor. That of course was not where the story ended. The world is so obsessed with sex that it demands that everyone be identified by a sexual label. Everyone must be included for this ideology to work, otherwise this notion of "sexual equality" crumbles. So what about the people in the middle, the ones who are sexually attracted to both genders? Where does their "sexual orientation" point? Somewhere along the line "bisexual" was the "sexual identity" invented to accommodate those individuals and the process continued. Now one would think there is a glaring flaw in this design: how can everyone have a "sexual orientation" and in turn a "sexual identity" when there are people who aren't sexually attracted to anyone? This is a fantastic question. The answer, however, is outlandish: these individuals do have a "sexual orientation" and their "sexual identity" is "asexual." Did you catch that? Remember, for this ideology to work no group of people can be left out, so a "sexual identity" was invented to label those who aren't sexually attracted to anyone. In other words, their "sexual identity" is they don't have a "sexual identity." This pattern of inventing "sexual identities" on a whim continues to this day. If everyone has a "sexual orientation" and that "sexual orientation" determines everyone's "sexual identity" then there has to be a name for those "sexual identities." To my amazement the current list of terms and possible "sexual identities" has increased to over thirty and with every new sexual attraction/behavior that's not on the list, another label is simply invented and added. They've even invented a "sexual identity" for those who aren't sure what their sexual preferences are yet. They are called "questioning" and are encouraged to keep spinning the "sexual orientation" dial and keep experimenting wherever it lands until they figure it out.

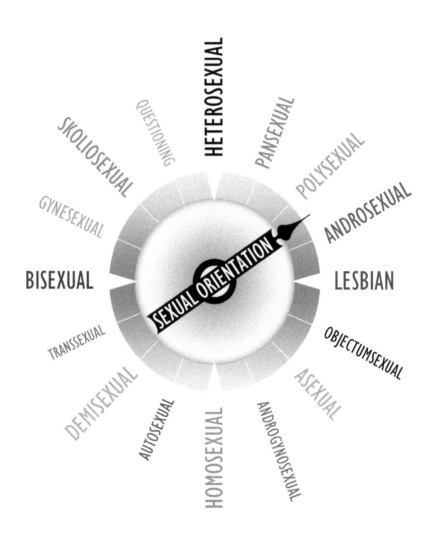

**FIGURE 1**
The "Sexual Orientation" Dial

There's an excellent chance that you've never seen many of the "sexual identities" on this graphic (Figure 1), which means you don't know what they mean. I most certainly didn't prior to my research. To show you how ridiculous this concept of "sexuality identity" has become, I'll provide a few definitions for you:

> *Autosexual* – an individual who is sexually attracted to him/herself and/or prefers masturbation to sex.
> *Objectumsexual* – an individual who is sexually attracted to inanimate objects.
> *Skoliosexual* – an individual who is sexually attracted to genderqueer or non-binary people.

Can you see the foolishness in this? People are literally indulging in all sorts of bizarre sexual activity and then adopting invented "sexual identities" as if that is literally who they are. Moreover, the creation of all of these "sexual identities" has further shifted the focus away from the "heterosexual" versus "homosexual" controversy. Now the "heterosexual" identity is far outnumbered, which creates the illusion that heterosexuality isn't the normal one anymore. Now that it appears to be in the minority (even though it isn't), *all* "sexual identities" have become the new normal. Of course, anyone who denies this illusory mindset is chastised as hateful and intolerant, while those who wholeheartedly embrace the fantasy are loving and tolerant.

# Americans Drastically Overestimate the "LGBT" Population in America

By creating the false reality that "homosexuals" make up a significant percentage of society, many people add credence to homosexuality as a valid and approved lifestyle. The truth, however, is the numbers are not nearly as high as most presume. This says quite a bit about homosexuality and the effective strategy "LGBT" activists have implemented to manipulate our perception. According to the latest polls[3] the average American estimate is twenty-three percent of the population are "homosexuals." Many estimate much higher percentages. I heard a man suggest "homosexuals" make up half the U.S. population. The fact is these estimates are well beyond the actual number, which is slightly above three and a half percent. This is highly significant when examining homosexuality. "LGBT" activists are well aware the higher the percentage of "homosexuals," the more support they garner and the more powerful the "gay movement" becomes. There is strength in numbers after all and their strategy has been to increase this low percentage in a number of devious ways, while convincing everybody that the percentage is already much higher than it is.

## All Homosexuals are Not United

Another fallacy perpetrated by "LGBT" activists is that the "LGBT" community is united on "homosexual" issues. They've fabricated this "us versus them" mentality where all homosexuals and advocates are on one team and everyone else is on the opposing team. This couldn't be further from the truth. The fact is that "homosexuals" are as divided as any other group, which is one of the reasons homosexuality is such a controversial issue. There are untold "homosexuals" who believe that homosexuality is not normal, natural, moral, or healthy. Some do not believe God approves of homosexuality. Some oppose "gay marriage" and same-sex parenting. Some do not believe "homosexuals" are born that way. Some believe the right course of action is to reject SSA, to refrain from and discourage homosexuality instead of promoting, defending, and indulging in it. The reality is that there is no consensus among "homosexuals." They struggle with these issues and debate them amongst each other.

Many practicing "homosexuals" appear to fully embrace homosexuality on the surface but deep down they are utterly conflicted by it. Take Pastor DL Foster for example. Pastor Foster is a prominent "ex-gay" activist who has been free from homosexuality for over twenty-five years now. I had the pleasure of speaking with him and one of the things that stuck with me from our conversation was that through all the years of indulging in homosexuality, he said in his heart of hearts he knew it was wrong. There are countless others who feel the same way, which contradicts the notion that all "homosexuals" believe homosexuality is moral.

There are even "gay" celebrities who are bold enough to share their conflicting views. In a candid interview, celebrity fitness trainer Jillian Michaels, who identifies as a "lesbian," admitted that she's still uncomfortable with homosexuality, and that it would be a dream to be normal – which directly implies that homosexuality is abnormal. Celebrity designers Dolce and Gabbana, who are both "gay," are vehemently opposed to "gay marriage" and same-sex parenting and have spoken out against both for many years. So what happens when members of the "LGBT" community publicly express these views that directly oppose the "homosexual" movement? One would think the "tolerant" advocates and "LGBT" activists would say, "We appreciate your viewpoint, which is as valid as ours." This is not the case at all. Even the homosexuals who oppose homosexuality are immediately demonized, boycotted, and ostracized from the "LGBT" community. This sort of treatment is more akin to a cult than a community, but this remains a little-known fact.

## "LGBT" Activists Lied – They Have Been Recruiting Children

Iconic superheroes in comics are now starting to "come out" as "gay." Now while that may seem miniscule to those who don't care about comic books, it is not miniscule at all. Consider how many kids are obsessed with superheroes and how much they want to dress like them, and act like them because they imagine how incredible it would be to actually *be* them. Now imagine how kids will respond to reading a comic book where their favorite superhero announces he or she is "gay." I was a comic book collector as a child, and I can only imagine how powerful and confusing that experience would have been for me, but the objective is clear: if superheroes, the good guys who are constantly saving the world from evil, are "gay", then being "gay" must be a good thing. Of course, this strategy is not limited to comic books. Even popular cartoons on children's networks now include "homosexual" characters. Animated movies are no exception. It may surprise you to learn in the popular animated series, "How to Train Your Dragon," Gobber, the one-handed Viking who trains and looks after the kids, is a "homosexual" character.

I recently watched a video called "Kids React to Gay Marriage"[4] where a group of children were shown two videos (one of a man proposing to another man, and another of a woman proposing to another woman) in order to capture their reactions. Shock and confusion were paramount, but then the off-screen interviewer began asking the children biased questions that shaped their reactions. In the end the consensus of the group was: "It doesn't matter if a man marries and man or a woman marries a woman; people should be able to be with whomever they love."

Prior to the tolerance for homosexuality we see today, whenever someone suggested "LGBT" activists had a strategy to indoctrinate children those allegations were vehemently denied. In fact, I recently Googled "homosexuals recruit" and the majority of the top results were articles claiming that "homosexual" recruitment was merely a conspiracy theory, that these were nothing but false accusations, etc. A little further digging unveiled the truth. Now that the indoctrination has been in full swing for some time, and homosexuality is as popular as it is, "LGBT" advocates are admitting they have indeed been indoctrinating our children in order to strengthen their movement. Consider the following quotes:

**"LGBT" activist, Daniel Villarreal (vulgar language has been censored):**
*They accuse us of exploiting children and in response we say, "NOOO! We're not gonna make kids learn about homosexuality, we swear! It's not like we're trying to recruit your children or anything." But let's face it—that's a lie. We want educators to teach future generations of children to accept queer sexuality. In fact, our future depends on it. Why would we push anti-bullying programs or social studies classes that teach kids about the historical contributions of famous queers unless we wanted to deliberately educate children to accept queer sexuality as normal? I would very much like for many of these young boys to grow up and start [having sex with] men.*

41

*I want lots of young ladies to develop into young women who [have sex with women]. I and a lot of other people want to indoctrinate, recruit, teach, and expose children to queer sexuality AND THERE'S NOTHING WRONG WITH THAT.*[5]

## "LGBT" activist and "transgender man", Sason Bear Bergman:

*All that time I said I wasn't indoctrinating anyone with my beliefs about gay and lesbian and bi and trans and queer people? That was a lie. I want to make them like us. That is absolutely my goal. I want to make your children like people like me and my family, even if that goes against the way you have interpreted the teachings of your religion.*

What's most telling is this final quote on the targeted indoctrination of children in schools, which was written back in 1987.

## Homosexual Activist Michael Swift:

*"We shall seduce them in your schools ... They will be recast in our image. They will come to crave and adore us."*[6]

Perhaps you were unaware this indoctrination has been in full swing for some time now. The litany of secrets revealed in an article called "'Making Schools Safe' Means 'Refashioning Values' in Massachusetts[7] is enlightening, albeit disturbing. There are "LGBT" groups such as GLSEN (Gay/Lesbian and Straight Education Network) that are wholly dedicated to shaping the minds of children in favor of homosexuality. As such, they have designed promotional material, hosted exhibits, and held mandatory assemblies in middle and high schools across the nation to teach children about homosexuality. This is often done without the knowledge or consent of parents and is disguised by positive sounding themes such as "Anti-bullying." Groups such as GLSEN reason it is preferable for parents to have no input on whether or not their children should be exposed to homosexuality in school, because to deny a child this important information is a blatant act of discrimination against the "LGBT" community. Secondly, they believe it is wrong for parents to force their beliefs and values on their children. Instead, children should be afforded the opportunity to choose for themselves, which is hypocritical because these "LGBT" groups then force their beliefs and values on the children. To avoid allowing parents to spread their "anti-homosexual" ideas to their children, the parents are bypassed altogether. The children are taught homosexuality is normal and acceptable, and "homophobia" (a made-up term with a definition that has evolved to hatred of "homosexuals" or homosexuality) is a disease that their parents might suffer from. Of course, this is totally contradictory. How is it "wrong" for parents to instill their values in their own children, but it is "right" for advocates, who aren't even related to these children, to instill their values in them instead?

There is actually an event called "anti-homophobia week," where a series of workshops, seminars, and lessons are conducted in classes. "Gays", "lesbians", and "transgenders" are brought into schools to speak to the children about their respective lifestyles and the goals they wish to achieve, such as being able to get married and adopt children. The "homosexual" agenda is pushed throughout this entire week, and young children are actually taught things such as oral and anal sex are normal and preferable, as neither result in pregnancy.

In one classroom lesson on discrimination, the children were made to perform a play and were given roles as "homosexuals." Boys were paired with boys and girls with girls. They were given lines to recite about the normalcy of homosexuality and the desire to be accepted and were then made to act out their roles as "homosexual" couples.

An abundance of surveys are given out at these events that include pointed questions about the children's "sexual orientation"—mind you, these are middle schools and high schools. Surveys included questions such as:

- Is it possible that heterosexuality is a phase you will grow out of?
- If you've never slept with anyone of the same sex, how do you know you wouldn't prefer it?
- Is it possible you need a good gay experience?

The children who are confused by these questions are taken into private sessions with "homosexual" counselors to discuss the child's sexuality. Historically, girls who would have fallen into the category of "tomboys" are now taught they are transgender and are also taken to special counselors to learn about their condition, once again without parental knowledge or consent.

History, health, science, and biology classes, along with sex education lessons, have now been redesigned with a special focus on introducing and promoting homosexuality. Dr. Michael Brown recounts:

> *While I was speaking at a Christian leader's gathering in Queens, New York, a pastor told the group that his son, also in high school, came home from his sex-ed class with some upsetting news. One of the students asked the teacher, "How do you know if you're gay?" and the teacher responded, "You should try it out for a month and see."*[8]

This was to a kid in high school. What's even more alarming is they have even produced books for children in kindergarten and elementary schools that promote homosexuality so by the time these children reach middle school it will be even easier to mold them into advocates if they aren't already. In Lexington, Massachusetts, children were given copies of a picture book called *Who's in a Family?* and were told same-sex couples are another kind of family, like their own parents.[9]

This contradictory trend continues in the homes of many same-sex couples. Same-sex couples would obviously desire to raise children to be advocates of homosexuality at the least; however, the objective of many same-sex couples is to raise their children to actually be "homosexuals." Of course, those in same-sex relationships who are raising children rarely admit this, as again, it is a blatant contradiction, but there are some who unashamedly admit the truth. Take CNN political commentator Sally Kohn, for instance. Sally freely admitted her intentions in her article in *The Washington Post* titled, "I'm gay. And I want my kid to be gay, too."[10] What's interesting is Sally contradicts herself multiple times in her article, saying on one hand, "No matter what, I'd want my child to be herself," then a few paragraphs later she admits:

> *We've bought every picture book featuring gay families, even the not-very-good ones, and we have most of the nontraditional-gender-role books as well—about the princess who likes to fight dragons, and the boy who likes to wear dresses. When my daughter plays house with her stuffed koala bears as the mom and dad, we gently remind her that they could be a dad and a dad.*

That's not letting her child "be herself" at all. It's brainwashing disguised as something innocent. It is also an excellent example of how the "LGBT" ideology is being fed to our impressionable-minded youth and rationalized as though it is acceptable moral practice.

Are you noticing a trend? There is a dedicated initiative focused solely on training today's youth to approve of homosexuality. It is a fundamental component of a movement to force a major change in our society. Remember, the goal is a reformed society where homosexuality (and other practices that are commonly seen as taboo) are no longer frowned upon, but are embraced, encouraged, and celebrated. The only successful method of forcing a fundamental change in a society is the relentless targeting of every demographic with a particular focus on the youngest minds in that society. Why? Because the youngest minds are the most impressionable — their minds are the easiest to mold. So once an entire young generation is convinced there is nothing wrong with homosexuality, it will only be a matter of time before the vast majority of society are advocates or "homosexuals", and the shift will be completed.

## Mainstream Media is Dedicated to Promoting Homosexuality

Total media domination was essential in advancing the "gay rights" movement. To ensure this happened, "homosexuals" and advocates implemented a brilliant master plan where individuals were strategically positioned in organizations and institutions (most often in the government and mainstream media), where they quietly advanced until they held positions of power and were free to push the "homosexual" agenda. This continues even now. For years one of the "LGBT" activists' primary objectives has been to add "homosexual" characters and themes to every major TV show in order to make them more "inclusive." Today we can all see how successful this campaign has been. It was a gradual process that began with shows including "homosexual" hints, subtle references, and "homosexual" humor, all in small doses to desensitize viewers to what was really happening. Next, shows would simply introduce "homosexual" characters in secondary roles. As time passed, "homosexual" characters became more prominent, they were given primary roles, and then they were shown dating and kissing members of the same sex. Today they have gone even further and have begun actually showing gay sex scenes on primetime TV shows. The time for hints or subtle references is long gone. Now, homosexuality is so prevalent that it's difficult to find a current TV show that does not include it.

## Homosexuals are Extremely Promiscuous

The incredibly high level of promiscuity in the "homosexual" community is also a little known fact that "LGBT" activists want to keep secret. Dr. Thomas Schmidt in his book *Straight and Narrow?* says, "Promiscuity among homosexual men is not a mere stereotype, and it is not merely the majority experience—it is virtually the *only* experience . . . lifelong faithfulness is almost non-existent in the homosexual experience."[11] "Homosexual" couple David McWhirter and Andrew Mattison even corroborate this fact in their book *The Male Couple: How Relationships Develop*. The authors detail a study of 156 committed "homosexual" male couples. The results of the study were that of the 100+ couples that endured beyond five years, not a single one had been sexually monogamous or exclusive. McWhirter and Mattison argued that, for male couples, sexual monogamy is a passing stage of internalized homophobia and that what matters for male couples is emotional, not physical, faithfulness.[12] Pastor DL Foster also corroborates this fact from his personal experience. He explained the term "committed relationship" means something entirely different in the "homosexual" community. While committed "heterosexual" relationships prohibit infidelity, there is no such prohibition in "homosexual" relationships. In fact, Pastor Foster explained how he used to purposely pursue men in "committed relationships" and was never once turned away because the "gay" men he pursued were spoken for. In the "homosexual community" it is simply common practice to have no sexual restrictions, even for those in "committed relationships." So in other words, they have their cake and eat it too. You can only imagine the level of promiscuity this unwritten rule encourages. In an astonishing study of 2,583 older "homosexuals" published in *Journal of Sex Research,* Paul Van de Ven, et al., discovered the median range of lifetime sexual partners was between 101–500. Beyond that, 10.2 percent to 15.7 percent of the men studied had between 501 and 1000 partners, while a further 10.2 percent to 15.7 percent of the men had more than 1000 lifetime sexual partners.[13] In ordinary circumstances, if someone has had hundreds to over a thousand sexual partners, they are vilified and called all sorts of foul names for being so promiscuous. In order to keep this from happening in the "homosexual" community, revealing information like this is kept a secret at all costs. It's also a little-known fact that there are all sorts of ways in which "homosexual" promiscuity is facilitated. There are actually mobile apps that allow "homosexuals" to search the profiles of other "homosexuals" (wherever they happen to be) to hook up and have sex—even with total strangers. So appeasing the homosexually promiscuous is now as easy as using a mobile app.

# Terry Bean was Arrested for Sexual Abuse and Sodomy Charges Against a Fifteen-year-old Boy

There are dozens of "LGBT" activist groups in operation today. Among the most popular are GLAAD (Gay & Lesbian Alliance Against Defamation), NOH8 Campaign, and the Human Rights Campaign (HRC). These groups are well funded, they work tirelessly to promote and defend the "gay" agenda, and they push their agenda behind the mask of love, equality, inclusion, and tolerance. However, their approach is not always peaceful. The HRC, for example, is known for going on the attack against high-profile individuals who publicly declare their disapproval of homosexuality and work to preserve the sanctity of marriage and family. The HRC "exposes" these individuals and brands them "extremists" and "bigots," describing them with words such as "vicious," "venomous," and "hateful." They even claim these individuals and their organizations put the lives of the "LGBT" community at risk. Essentially, the picture they paint is: "These are the names and faces of the individuals who hate us and are threatening our lives." Why do they do this? To incite a furious response. The response has come in the form of hate mail, insults, attacks, lawsuits, and death threats, which are ironically all *hateful*. What most people don't know is Terry Bean, the sixty-six-year-old cofounder of the HRC (and friend and major supporter of Barack Obama), was arrested along with his twenty-five-year-old boyfriend for allegedly raping a fifteen-year-old boy.[14] The founder and champion of one of the largest and most prominent "LGBT" rights organizations, who has painted opposers as immoral, is secretly involved in truly immoral behavior.

Although Bean maintains his innocence, the fact is, the testimony of the fifteen-year-old victim perfectly matched the account of Bean's boyfriend in describing the sexual encounter between the two men and the young teen. Bean has argued he wasn't even there, but financial records prove it was he who paid for the hotel room. Bean attempted to settle the case by paying off his victim, but settling a sexual assault case with a minor is unprecedented so the judge rejected Bean's deal. This immediately raises the question: why was Terry Bean willing to offer over $200,000 and more undisclosed incentives to settle the case if he was indeed innocent? Bean's excuse was that this case was damaging his reputation and well-being by possibly worsening the condition of his prostate cancer, which has reportedly spread. Nevertheless, right when it looked like the writing was on the wall, the case was ultimately dismissed. Apparently the victim was too distraught and uncomfortable describing their three-way sexual encounter in front of the media and a courtroom full of people. This sudden reversal in the victim's willingness to testify is a red flag that has many convinced that there was a secret payoff to keep him quiet. Bean of course claims this is proof that he is totally innocent, but this is contrary to the sworn testimony of both the victim and Bean's then boyfriend. The victim has maintained his sworn testimony is factual and never wavered from his story, which speaks volumes. So while the charges against Bean were dismissed, they were dismissed without prejudice, which means the charges can be filed again. Time will tell if the victim changes his mind and decides to testify so that justice will be done.

In the midst of this fiasco, another victim boldly stepped forward, who was sixteen when Bean provided him with alcohol, drugs, and had a sexual relationship with him. In addition to that, the investigation into Bean's sexual activity with minors is ongoing. As we wait to see how this little-publicized story develops, I wonder how many people know the graphic of an equal sign that they stick on their cars and post online is actually the HRC logo. I wonder how those people would react if they knew the sexually deviant behavior of the HRC's founder whom they are unwittingly promoting.

## Christians are Targeted and Persecuted Simply Because of their Faith

Arguably the greatest line of defense against the global domination of the "homosexual" movement is Christianity. This is why a considerable amount of the "LGBT" proponents have focused on attacking Christians and the church. Homosexuality, marriage, love, and purity—these are all topics found in the Bible, and specific parameters and instructions have been established to distinguish between moral and immoral behavior. So what happens when the Bible says something people don't like? They could do some self-introspection and focus on *why* they dislike God's commands, but this appears to be an unpopular response. The most common options are to try to change what God's Word says, or to ignore God's commands altogether by denouncing the Bible, God, and Christianity. Those who attempt to change what God's Word says attend "LGBT" friendly churches where practicing "homosexuals" are encouraged and some pastors are even practicing "homosexuals" themselves. They claim the Bible can be interpreted in many ways, followed by the claim that their interpretation of the Bible does not condemn homosexuality. They then conclude they are free to be practicing "homosexual Christians."

Even religious courses in colleges and universities have taken a more "progressive" stance. Professors often present slanted versions of Christianity, teaching what they *wish* the Bible says instead of what it *actually* says in order to promote homosexuality. Those who ignore God's commands altogether often become agnostics (those who claim they don't know if God exists) or atheists (those who believe or claim God does not exist) in order to eliminate any moral accountability. They claim Christians are hateful, bigoted fools for believing in a God who doesn't exist and for standing on the principles of an ancient book full of errors, contradictions, and fairytales. This smear campaign has also been fairly successful. To say, "I am a Christian," today is often met with eye rolls, and sighs, and disdainful looks. This was done by design.

Despite the will of the people, the Supreme Court has now ruled in favor of gay "marriage" nationwide, which means there are judges who are forced to comply and issue marriage licenses to same-sex couples. A number of Christian judges with long histories serving the judicial system have opted to step down rather than violate their religious beliefs by participating in "homosexual" unions.

Kim Davis, the county clerk of Rowan County, Kentucky, was jailed for six days after refusing to sign "gay marriage" licenses, and set a precedent as the first person jailed in the United States for holding to their Christian faith. Christian wedding photographers, florists, wedding planners, bakeries, and wedding chapels that refuse to violate their faith suffer detrimental consequences as well. We've seen a sudden flood of cases where "gay" couples were declined services by Christian-owned bakeries. This is not a coincidence. Many times this was done purposely and with the full knowledge that their request would be declined based on Christian beliefs. "Gay" couples targeted these bakeries with the express intent of suing them for "discrimination." As a result, we've seen an abundance of lawsuits, ranging in the hundreds of thousands of dollars, coupled with smear campaigns and boycotts that have destroyed businesses and devastated the lives of Christian business owners.

It isn't enough to simply go to a bakery that doesn't oppose "gay marriage" to achieve the goal of getting married.

No, this is done deliberately because the ultimate goal is not to get married, but to make it clear that if you oppose homosexuality, then you will be punished and punished severely. Is this practicing love, tolerance, and acceptance? Not at all. Apparently, the concept of love, tolerance, and acceptance in response to Christians is vengeance. Consequently, Christians continue to be sued, harassed, vilified, threatened, and attacked for choosing to honor their faith instead of compromising their moral principles. Religious freedom laws (although they are not new) suddenly became a polarizing hot-topic. Many proponents of homosexuality claim these laws foster and condone discrimination against *people*, while others understand these laws protect everyone's right to refuse to participate in an *activity* that violates one's faith. This distinction is lost on many, but fortunately there are individuals in the "LGBT" community who understand this and are in favor of these laws despite the overwhelming opposition of their peers.

This trend of enacting punishment on anyone who publicly opposes homosexuality appears to have kicked into high gear around the time that GLAAD incited A&E to punish *Duck Dynasty* star Phil Robertson for making "anti-homosexual" comments. Robertson merely responded to a question regarding his definition of sin and gave an answer based on Scripture. Robertson then suffered the wrath of advocates and the "LGBT" community. A&E suspended him "indefinitely" and the future of the show was in jeopardy. If it wasn't for the public outcry in Robertson's defense, A&E would never have relented and allowed Robertson to continue filming his show. Nevertheless, the statement was made and with that precedent set, there's been a snowball effect.

Openly gay Houston mayor Annise Parker actually subpoenaed the sermons of five pastors in an effort to silence them from speaking against homosexuality. Fortunately, after the public once again rose in defense of the pastors, the subpoenas were dropped. Mozilla CEO Brendan Eich was forced to resign after making a donation to opponents of "gay marriage." Christian twins David and Jason Benham were set to host an HGTV show called *Flip it Forward,* but the show was pulled before it ever aired because the twins openly oppose homosexuality and abortion. Chaplains and ministers volunteering in the community and military are being given ultimatums to either agree to stop speaking out against homosexuality, or lose their positions. Many have opted to give up their positions to maintain their faith. Pastors are being pressured to marry "gay" couples even if they are opposed to "gay marriage", and "LBGT" activists are working diligently to end the tax-exempt status of religious institutions as punishment for their biblical views. Christianity is under attack. Reports of individuals being punished for their Christian faith are coming out more frequently and are showing no sign of slowing down.

# Next Steps

I could go on and on, but I believe the "LGBT" activists' end goal and the methodology to reach their goal has been made quite clear. Under the rainbow banner of love, tolerance, and equality, there is diabolical hypocrisy. At the core of the "gay rights" movement is an ideology and methodology that says, "if you agree with us then we love you and are tolerant of you, but if you disagree with us then we're allowed to hate you and be intolerant of you." This proves the quest for equality is a farce because equality says, "we're equal even if we disagree," but that's not at all what "LGBT" activists believe. They believe they are superior to those opposed to homosexuality, and are justified in exacting vengeance against any opposition. The true objective is not love, tolerance, and equality; the true objective is sexual freedom through the elimination of all opposition. In summary, the proactive strategy of the "gay rights" movement is essentially:

- To further the "gay" agenda through lies and deception if necessary.
- Incite anger by negatively labeling opposers with words such as hateful, homophobe, bigot, and intolerant.
- Incite compassion by positively labeling homosexuality with words such as loving, equality, natural, normal, and tolerant.
- Hide/ignore all negative aspects of homosexuality.
- Incite sympathy by labeling "homosexuals" as innocent victims who need to be defended.
- Incite vengeance by labeling opposers as bullies who need to be confronted and punished.
- Incite antitheism by labeling God, the Bible, and Christianity old fashioned, false, and foolish.
- Force change through repetition and constant inundation of "LGBT" ideology through every possible outlet: government, media, schools, corporations, etc.
- Force change by avoiding parents and interacting directly with children.
- Publicly praise all allies and supporters of homosexuality.
- Publicly shame and attack all opposers of homosexuality.

How are we to respond to these facts? Firstly we have to acknowledge that homosexuality is not limited to our individual experiences. It's not just something that exists; it's a pervasive network. It's like a living organism that continues to grow and spread and has a specific purpose: to be normalized in today's society and to redefine morality in the process. Secondly, we have to change this idea that remaining silent is a solution. This is precisely what "LGBT" activists want because they are well aware that silence actually aids them in enforcing their agenda.

In the beginning the objective of the "LGBT" community was tolerance—they simply wanted to be left alone to live as they pleased without disruption or persecution. Now their primary objective is universal acceptance, and to achieve this they aim to either convert everyone who disagrees or, at the least, render them silent. Does a monumental issue like homosexuality with repercussions of such magnitude warrant silence? Again, remaining silent certainly is easier and safer than speaking up, but is that the right option? Today many Christian pastors reason that if they speak out against homosexuality, their advocate church members will be offended and leave the church, which means a smaller congregation and less tithes and offering. On the other hand, they reason if they speak out in favor of homosexuality, their anti-homosexual church members will be offended and leave the church, which means a smaller congregation and less tithes and offering. Therefore, to avoid offending anyone and risking anyone leaving and taking their money with them, these pastors carefully avoid the issue entirely. I've been a Christian nearly my entire life, I've been to countless church services all over the country, and I've only heard one message on homosexuality beyond the one I delivered myself. This shouldn't be the case.

Many Christians admittedly also take the safe and easy route. Several people I know have confessed they purposely avoid the issue of homosexuality because they don't want to wind up in an argument. Of course, the question that follows is, how does remaining silent help anyone or change anything? It doesn't. So as Christians we must understand exactly what is going on and we must speak the truth in love despite the cultural shift to embrace homosexuality.

## The Best Approach to Homosexuality

As with anything else, if we approach the matter of homosexuality from the wrong perspective, we will come away with inaccurate conclusions. In my experience, most people who have made up their minds and planted their feet in favor of homosexuality approach the topic from a biological, political, or emotional standpoint. Those who take the biological route argue homosexuality is natural. "Homosexuals are born that way," they say. "It's not something that can be changed or cured." The arguments of those who take the political route are often centered on topics such as human rights, discrimination, and "marriage equality." Those who take the emotional route say things such as, "we should just love everyone, not hate," "everyone should be tolerant," "live and let live," and, "love is love." The question that remains is, which of these, if any, is the best approach to homosexuality? If none of the aforementioned qualifies, then the conclusions people have reached based on those approaches are most likely inaccurate.

When it comes to matters of intellect, I've found emotionally charged approaches are insufficient as they often lead us astray. In fact, it's quite dangerous to abandon thought and rely on feelings alone. Given this, we cannot afford to use our feelings to tackle this difficult subject, and so we will not. The best approach to homosexuality is a rational, logical approach from a moral perspective. Now what do I mean by rational? Rational means clear thinking based on *facts* and *reason,* not on opinions and feelings. Conversely, irrational means unclear thinking based on *opinions* and *feelings,* not on facts and reason. I'll give you a couple examples. I'm sure like me, you are guilty of making an impulse buy at some point. You walked through a store with absolutely no intention of buying a certain item, but that item caught your eye and suddenly you felt the urge to buy it.

Now in those situations your rational brain says things such as, "We can't afford this right now. This is not something we need. Keep walking and get what you came in here for."

Your irrational brain on the other hand counters and says, "But we want it. It's on sale. We can just charge it and worry about paying for it later."

Then you say, "Okay!" You buy it and then suffer from putting yourself deeper in debt. That's an irrational decision.

Another example, one I've also been guilty of many times, concerns dating. My rational brain says, "I'm not compatible with her. We don't have good conversations. I don't even like her that much."

My irrational brain says, "She's cute though. So date her."

Then I say, "Okay!" I date her and waste time, energy, and money, and then we wind up breaking up because we were never compatible in the first place. So what can we learn from these examples? Wisdom says to be rational and avoid irrationality. That's precisely what we will do here regarding homosexuality.

Now logic is the proper, systematic method of thinking to reach accurate conclusions. Illogic, then, is using an improper method of thinking, which results in reaching inaccurate conclusions. Our goal is to only reach accurate conclusions on homosexuality, so to ensure this happens we must use logic.

Now why are we looking at homosexuality from a moral perspective? Homosexuality is, above all else, a moral issue. Morality is the primary objective for all humans; we're all obligated to be moral individuals. So people can argue all day long about whether "homosexuals" are born that way or choose to be that way, or whether or not "homosexuals" should be allowed to marry, or whether "homosexuals" should be allowed to adopt children, but in the end, the question of morality still remains. If homosexuality is immoral at its core, the rest of those things simply don't matter. So regardless what the Supreme Court rules or anyone feels, if homosexuality is immoral, then it shouldn't be practiced. This leads us to the first and most critical question that we must answer: *Is homosexuality sinful?* We will closely examine this question in the following chapters.

# 2

## Is Homosexuality Sinful?
## The "No" Position (I)

Is homosexuality sinful? This is a "yes or no" question. Once again, there are those (even professing Christians) who passionately answer, "No!" Then there are others who passionately answer, "Yes!" Homosexuality cannot be both sinful and not sinful, so the answer is clearly either "yes" or it is "no." To my great astonishment, I discovered there is actually a third answer. I visited a friend's church and met their pastor. "Pastor Chris" had "gay" members in his church and appeared to condone homosexuality based on a blog entry he posted online titled, "Tips on being straight/gay in church." I was shocked by the title and read his blog entry with great curiosity. Sadly, I found its content unsettling. Pastor Chris essentially compared two couples—one "gay," and one "straight." He concluded the individuals in both couples were all friendly Christians, and his life and his church were better with them in it, which makes the couples equal.

This left me perplexed, so I asked Pastor Chris: "Is homosexuality sinful?"

After a lengthy dissertation, he finally answered the question by saying: "I don't know." Not "Yes," not "No," but, "I don't know." He said he knows what the Bible says, and he understands the Scripture, but he simply couldn't bring himself to say that homosexuality was sinful. He claimed the issue was too complex to be certain, so instead of committing to a firm answer he simply chooses to say, "I don't know."

Later I discovered the blog I'd read was a revised version of the original, which introduced his "I don't know" position a year prior. Reading the lengthier original was also disturbing. Pastor Chris explained how potential church members asked about his position on the "LGBT" community and he replied saying, "I don't know." He told them that if they were okay with that, then he would love to have them at his church. This resulted in a significant number of "gays" and "lesbians" visiting and joining his congregation. In fact, Pastor Chris told me the majority of the members in his congregation were practicing "gays" and "lesbians." Now this is the part that blew my mind. He told me every single one of them struggles with homosexuality. Every single one has come to him privately and confessed they struggle with this lifestyle and looked to him for guidance.

The fact that they all struggle with homosexuality is an excellent sign. That means that there is an internal problem that needs to be fixed, and they can't be comfortable or at peace until that happens. You know what he told them all? He said, "I don't know." Can you believe that?

"You're a pastor," I told him. "People come to you for help—that's what pastors are for, and you're telling them 'I don't know'? That's unacceptable because it is your job to know. How can you help anyone by not knowing?" I reminded him that he is in an awesome position; he has an incredible opportunity to help people and save lives. Sadly, it was like talking to brick wall. I then asked him how long he planned on maintaining a neutral position of ignorance withholding the answers his congregation comes to him for? Of course, he didn't know the answer to that either.

We continued to debate the issue, but nothing changed, and although he encouraged me to keep challenging him, he abandoned the conversation soon afterward. After nearly a year of silence, I decided to find out if anything had changed. Mind you, the first blog entry was written in January 2013, the second in January of 2014, and here it was nearly January of 2015 when I reached out and asked him if he finally settled on a position. I was saddened but not surprised to learn nothing had changed. After two full years Pastor Chris told me that he'd had many more conversations and read many more books but still didn't know if homosexuality was sinful. Pastor Chris actually admitted that a member of his church suffers from multiple STDs, including AIDS, and yet Pastor Chris still refuses to tell him or anyone else the truth about homosexuality. This man is *literally dying* as a result of homosexuality and Pastor Chris still never changed his neutral position. I then came to the conclusion that Pastor Chris either refuses to take a firm position on the matter for fear of losing church members, or he simply doesn't want to believe what he admittedly knows the Bible says about homosexuality, and so he simply avoids the truth. This is unacceptable for a true Christian pastor. Pastors are responsible for their flock, and God will judge any pastor harshly for leading their flock astray, but here's the good news: we don't have to spend years in "I don't know" limbo like Pastor Chris. We *can* know if homosexuality is sinful, and we can help others to know too. So let us apply ration and logic to this question to actually come to a real conclusion one way or the other.

In order to make matters perfectly clear, we need to fully understand the question being asked. We've already established homosexuality is erotic behavior with members of the same gender. Now what is sin? Sin is a willful violation of God's Moral Law. So the question, *Is homosexuality sinful?* translates to: *Is erotic behavior with members of the same gender a willful violation of God's Moral Law?* We will first consider the answer "No," and explore the reasons or arguments used to substantiate that answer. I've had a great number of discussions and debates on this issue with men and women, Christians and non-Christians, "homosexuals" and "heterosexuals," and when it comes to determining the moral status of homosexuality, I've noticed a number of common trends. Below are the top ten reasons or supporting arguments I've heard most often from those who claim homosexuality is not sinful.

1. "Who are you to judge?"
2. "You're just a hateful, homophobic, intolerant, bigot."
3. "They're the most loving and caring people I know."
4. "Why do you even care? How are they bothering you?"
5. "Everyone is equal."
6. "You should just love everyone and treat everyone with kindness."
7. "There's nothing wrong with people who are in love being together."
8. "They're born that way."
9. "Jesus never spoke against homosexuality."
10. "The Scriptures against homosexuality have been misinterpreted/mistranslated."

Now the first question we should ask ourselves in response to these popular arguments is: are any of these (individually or collectively) rational, logical premises that prove homosexuality is *not* sinful? The answer is a resounding *no,* and here's why. A logical fallacy is simply an error in reasoning. A fallacy is simply a false notion or belief. Every single one of these arguments commits at least one logical fallacy or is a fallacy in itself. Recall the question that was posed: is homosexuality sinful? In order to prove the illogical nature of these arguments, all one must do is add, "Therefore homosexuality is not sinful" at the end of each one. So the first becomes: "Who are you to judge? Therefore homosexuality is not sinful." This obviously makes no sense. This can be done with every single one of these, and you can clearly see none of these arguments are rational or logically sound. Nevertheless, let's take a closer look at each one and further explore their illogical nature.

### 1. "Who are you to judge?"

*Logical Fallacy Committed: Appeal to Hypocrisy*—avoiding the issue by answering criticism with criticism.

This is far and away the response I hear the most regarding homosexuality's moral status, but it's logically fallacious because it focuses on *criticizing* the claim that homosexuality is sinful instead of focusing on *proving* the claim that homosexuality is not sinful. This response also comes in various forms: "That's between them and God," "Only God can judge," "You don't have the right to judge," but they each imply the same thing: to make the claim that homosexuality is sinful is judging, and judging is something no one is permitted to do. Is this an accurate assessment? More importantly, does this adequately support the answer to the question at hand? No and no.

I've heard this "don't judge" comment so often I began to respond by asking, "What does that mean?" To my surprise, those who are so quick to tell me (and others) not to judge find it difficult to explain what they mean by that. It sounds quite foolish to imply it's wrong to state something is wrong because that is totally self-contradictory. Further, and most ironically, to say, "don't judge" is actually a judgment! It's judging that someone is being judgmental, and it is judging that they are making a wrong judgment. So it is quite hypocritical to go around telling others "don't judge." So what do people actually mean when they say, "Don't judge," to someone who opposes homosexuality? No one wants to come out and say it, but what they're actually implying by "don't judge," is "don't worry if what they're doing is right or wrong; be quiet and leave them alone." Once again, this does nothing to establish the moral status of homosexuality.

I was actually discussing homosexuality with a Christian friend of mine who is admittedly judgmental, and to my astonishment her response to me was that I shouldn't judge. I then explained the fact that identifying sinfulness is not "judging someone," and I reminded her that she is admittedly judgmental of others. She agreed, admitted that being judgmental was one of her character flaws, and backed off of that response. In another discussion with another Christian friend, the way she defined "not judging" was essentially to remain silent. I then submitted Jesus never remained silent in the face of sin, nor did His disciples, so why should we? She too began to backtrack, as she couldn't find any ground to stand on in response to what she knew to be true. As a Christian she too had a responsibility to help others by identifying sin, but she didn't like that idea when it came to homosexuality, so she simply ended the discussion.

So where does this whole confused and customized concept of "don't judge" come from? It's actually a quote from a sermon delivered by Jesus Christ Himself as recorded in the seventh chapter of Matthew. People who know this believe it adds more credibility to this overly quoted, frequently misunderstood Scripture. I watched a reality show where three couples went on vacation together, one of which was a "gay" couple. A Christian began to ask the gay couple questions. He explained that he'd been brought up in the church, and that according to the Bible homosexuality was wrong. Immediately, the other Christian couple responded with, "don't judge." One of the "gay" men, however, was happy to respond to the man's questions. He explained he too has a personal relationship with God, and therefore his lifestyle couldn't be challenged.

"Do not judge or you too will be judged," the "gay" man said, "and that's Matthew chapter seven."

To this the other couple said, "Amen!" and applauded him for his response. One praised him for seeming to know the Bible better than the Christian who posed the question, and then condoned her friends' "homosexual" lifestyle by asserting it's okay because they're born that way. It was unfortunate that not only did all the Christians in the room not see the glaring error in taking the Scripture out of context, but none of them had the wherewithal to offer an intelligent response based on the full passage of Matthew 7 balanced with the rest of Scripture. And so, in that setting, and on national TV, the message was: "Don't worry if what 'homosexuals' are doing is right or wrong; be quiet and leave them alone." This is the goal that many practicing "homosexuals" and advocates strive for, which is why they frequently quote Matthew 7 and lay it down like a "Get out of Hell Free" card. In essence, once "do not judge" is quoted from the Bible, they feel they're free to continue indulging in homosexuality without question or opposition. This is clearly fallacious and a distortion of the Scripture. When dealing with the Bible, we can never pluck out a single passage and frame it to mean something contrary to the full context of the passage and the Bible as a whole. So let's examine the text in context and see what Jesus is truly saying.

> Do not judge, or you too will be judged. For in the same way you judge others, you will be judged, and with the measure you use, it will be measured to you. Why do you look at the speck of sawdust in your brother's eye and pay no attention to the plank in your own

eye? How can you say to your brother, "Let me take the speck out of your eye," when all the time there is a plank in your own eye? You hypocrite, first take the plank out of your own eye, and then you will see clearly to remove the speck from your brother's eye (Matthew 7:1–6).

Notice how the full context of this passage is ignored. Jesus was not saying, "Be silent, and don't point out your brother's sin because you have way more sin than he does." No, there is a good kind of judging in Scripture and a bad kind of judging. The difference is the *purpose* and *nature* of the judging. In this example of bad judging, Jesus was exposing hypocrites who wished to go around being self-righteous by pointing out the sins in others, all while ignoring their greater quantity of sinfulness. Their purpose in judging was not to help restore their brothers but to win praise for *appearing* righteous, when in fact they were not. I'm sure you've witnessed people who go around telling on everyone else in order to make themselves look better. Jesus is forbidding this ridiculous behavior. His commandment was essentially: stop being hypocritical and turning a blind eye to your own sin while looking for sins in others. Stop living a sinful lifestyle—and this is the part that everyone leaves out—"then you will see clearly to remove the speck from your brother's eye." Notice Jesus didn't encourage anyone to *ignore* their brother's speck. The end goal was for both individuals to be free from sin and to live righteous lives. Therefore, simply saying, "Don't judge," does not justify or remove someone's speck. Furthermore, once Matthew 7 is taken in context, notice also what the other Scriptures say about judging. In John 7:21 Jesus says, "Stop judging by mere appearances and make a right judgment." The Apostle Paul says in 1 Corinthians 5:12, "Are you not to judge those inside [the church]?" This clearly shows "Do not judge" in Matthew 7 does not mean, "remain silent and excuse each other's sins," which is what many people are convinced it means. The purpose of good judging, which Christians are not only permitted to do but are obligated to do, is to help one another and save one another from sin.

In Luke 17:3 Jesus says, "If your brother sins, rebuke him, and if he repents forgive him." This obviously requires us to use judgment for the purpose of restoring our brother in Christ. So if I'm walking with my brother and he stumbles, my job is to help him and pick him back up. Likewise, if I stumble, my brother's job is to help me and pick me back up. That's the way the body of Christ functions. We look out for each other and help each other along the way because none of us are perfect. So now we can see even more clearly why "Do not judge" does absolutely nothing to justify homosexuality or prove homosexuality is not sinful.

**2. "You're just a hateful, homophobic, intolerant, bigot."**
*Logical Fallacy Committed: Ad hominem*—attacking the person instead of addressing the argument.

Where the previous logical fallacy avoids the issue and focuses on attacking any criticism to one's position, this logical fallacy avoids the issue and focuses on attacking the person instead. Of course this is not limited to the terms listed here. I've been called far more names, but the point remains that this tactic is not only disrespectful, it is logically fallacious. I don't believe it is right to attack anyone (verbally or otherwise) regardless of what position they take. This is critical because there are people who call themselves Christians who believe it is their right to attack "homosexuals," which is not Christ-like at all; it is clearly wrong. Then there are "homosexuals" and advocates who believe they have the right to attack Christians because they deserve it. This is also wrong.

Once again, attacking a person completely avoids the issue at hand.

What's even more ironic is many people who commit this logical fallacy also commit the previous one by saying, "Do not judge." I was engaged in an online discussion about how quickly people are these days to cry "hate" and "intolerance," which ironically is both hateful and intolerant. One of my friends joined the conversation with a wide ranging, angry argument about Christians being hateful, intolerant bigots who judge "homosexuals" and how horrible that was. I pointed out that not all Christians who oppose homosexuality are hateful or bigoted. True Christians love "homosexuals" and aren't condemning them, but are trying to save them. I then asked him how he could distinguish between the "Christians" he described and the Christians I described. He refused to answer my question because the answer was obvious and self-contradictory: he judges them! I found it fascinating that instead of acknowledging his own assessment was harsh, judgmental, and exactly what he accused Christians of doing to "homosexuals," he opted to simply not respond and held to his erroneous mindset. In fact, this happens more often than not concerning people and their position on homosexuality. Many people will make bold claims, call people names, and list everything that they consider to be wrong behavior based on their emotions and feelings (which is irrational), but when they're given a respectful, logical, and rational response that counters everything they've said and believe, they opt to simply dismiss it and continue in error. This is of course their prerogative, but it proves their goal is to hurl insults as a tactic to avoid admitting they are wrong instead of ascertaining and accepting the truth.

I had another conversation with an angry advocate who kept throwing out the word "intolerant," all while failing to see the self-contradictory nature of that accusation. The fact is that *everyone is intolerant*. I explained to him that those who point the finger at others and call them "intolerant" are actually being intolerant of those people. Nobody accepts everything, which renders the concept of universal tolerance preposterous. Once again, instead of an apology, or an acknowledgment that what I said was truthful, my rebuttal was met with utter silence. I then came to the conclusion that those who are quick to hurl insults and resort to name calling in situations like these are so driven by their feelings and opinions that they insist they are right regardless of how strong and factual the counterargument is. Instead of admitting fault, they will either continue to attack their opponents, or simply retreat without a word. Nevertheless, we have seen that committing *ad hominem* completely avoids the question of homosexuality's moral status and therefore totally fails to prove that homosexuality is not sinful.

**3. "They're the most loving and caring people I know."**
***Logical Fallacy Committed:*** *False Cause*—presuming a relationship between two things means one caused the other.

The thought behind this claim and those of similar nature is that "loving" and "caring" are clearly moral attributes, and since all the "homosexuals" a person knows exhibits those moral attributes, then homosexuality must also be moral behavior. Obviously this conclusion doesn't follow because a person's ability to be loving and caring is not a product of their homosexuality. One has absolutely nothing to do with the other. To make this clear, pick any immoral behavior you desire, put it in place of homosexuality in this formula, and see if it makes sense. I'll pick prostitution to show you what I mean: (Prostitutes) are the most loving and caring people I know; therefore, (prostitution) is moral behavior. As you can see, this is a completely illogical conclusion. A person's personality traits have nothing to do with the morality of their lifestyle. Personality traits don't override or excuse sinful behavior either. Like a prostitute with an incredible loving and caring disposition is not justified in prostitution because of that disposition, a "homosexual" with an incredibly loving and caring disposition is not justified in practicing homosexuality because of that disposition.

Further, to make the claim, "'Homosexuals' are the most loving and caring people I know" is actually a judgment. Isn't it interesting how that keeps showing up in these arguments? We've already established Jesus explicitly commanded us to not judge by mere appearances, and yet that is exactly what most people do. They cannot see inside a person's heart; they only see what they are shown, which can be anything from a facet of the truth to a total fabrication. This couldn't have been proven to me any better than the sobering story I read about a "homosexual" couple who everyone thought was loving and caring. A man named Mark Newton and his boyfriend Peter Truong bought a baby boy and called it an adoption. From the outside looking in, everything about this couple indicated they were loving and caring individuals who only wanted to have a family. Sadly this wasn't true. Behind closed doors they began to film themselves sexually abusing their "adopted" son, who at the time wasn't even two years old, and this continued until he was six years old. Then this "loving and caring" couple uploaded the footage of their unspeakable acts to a pedophilia network called Boy Lovers Network for other pedophiles to enjoy. To make matters even worse, Mark and Peter actually flew their "adopted" son around the world to allow other men to sexually abuse him while they filmed it. Even when these two were arrested and convicted (Newton was sentenced to forty and Truong to thirty years in prison), they showed no remorse nor did they consider their actions to be immoral. Mark Newton actually told the court, "Being a father was an honor and a privilege that amounted to the best six years of my life."[15] In a deceptive attempt to get away with their heinous crimes, Mark and Peter actually attempted to gain support by claiming they were discriminated against because they were "gay." Astonishingly the media picked up their story.

Detective Sergeant Ian Wells said Mark and Peter were master manipulators, using "gay marriage" as a cover. "For them to mount a media campaign and portray to their friends and neighbors and family that they're innocent individuals, it was sad," he said. "It was disgusting that they were willing to manipulate people close to them to try and get them on board, but that was them. They were manipulators; they were expert at it."[16]

This is the side of homosexuality that proponents of the lifestyle never talk about. They either consider it a rare extreme and ignore it, or they are oblivious to it altogether. Yet this is merely a glimpse of what goes on in the dark and behind closed doors in the "gay" community. The truth is to appear loving and caring does not make one loving and caring, nor does it justify one's immoral actions. Further, to actually love and care for others still does not justify one's immoral actions. Therefore this argument fails to prove homosexuality is not sinful.

**4. "Why do you even care? How are they bothering you?"**
*Logical Fallacy Committed: Red Herring*—introducing an irrelevant topic to shift attention away from the argument.

This response, while it may be a legitimate inquiry, is a distraction and does nothing to prove that homosexuality is moral. The "who cares?" response is one I've heard quite often and is simply an attempt to dissuade me from further discussing the topic. In my experience, the individuals who ask this question are passionate proponents of homosexuality and wish to simply avoid any opposition. To achieve this they attempt to make it seem foolish and even offensive to even broach the subject. However, remember this is a distraction to steer one away from dealing with the core issue. Nevertheless, I will answer the question. I care because I am a Christian. As a Christian my focus is not merely on *my* moral status and *my* eternal destination. I care about others and *their* moral status, and *their* eternal destination. It is not my desire for anyone to live an immoral lifestyle because it is damaging to themselves and to others. It is not my desire that anyone wind up suffering in torment for eternity for refusing to honor God to live an immoral lifestyle. I have been honored and blessed with opportunities to help other people by sharing my personal struggles with sexuality and explaining how I overcame them. I've encouraged virgins who struggled to maintain their sexual purity to remain virgins until marriage. I've encouraged sexually active individuals who desired to become celibate to overcome their sexual lifestyles. I've even helped practicing "homosexuals" on their path to recovery from their dangerous and addictive lifestyle. This is why I care.

Secondly, I must point out the motive behind the question, "How are they bothering you?" is deceiving. The real question being asked is: "If you just keep quiet and leave "homosexuals" alone, how does what they do affect your life?" Another popular phrase I often hear, which follows this line of thinking is: "Live and let live . . ." In other words: "They're leaving you alone, so leave them alone." Well, as I've already pointed out, there are militant gay activists who don't want to merely be left alone. They want to redefine morality, love, family, and sexual normalcy. They're targeting children along with every demographic from multiple angles. This "gay rights" movement doesn't just affect the "homosexual" community; it affects everyone. Their goal is to reshape our culture and change the fabric of our society. So just as sin bothers me, attempting to craft an entirely new society that accepts and promotes sin also bothers me. Any member of society has every right to stand against any threats to that society and uphold the purity of morality as defined by God. With that said, this type of distraction avoids the issue entirely and thus also fails as an argument to prove that homosexuality is not sinful.

**5. "Everyone is equal."**
***Logical Fallacy Committed:*** *False Equivalence*—claiming equivalence when in fact there is none.

"Equality" is a popular buzzword in the "gay rights" movement, and the claim "everyone is equal" more specifically implies "homosexuals" and "heterosexuals" are equal and should therefore be treated equally. It is easy to be pulled off track into a political discussion at this point, but let us remember the question we posed at the beginning: is homosexuality sinful? If it is not, then there could be validity to the concept of equality between "homosexuals" and "heterosexuals." If it is sinful, however, there is no such equality. I'll use a graphic I've often seen online to explain why. There's an image going around that shows identical skeletons standing side by side. Each skeleton is identified below with the words "black," "white," "gay," "straight," "religious," "atheist," and "you." At the top of this graphic in big letters is the word "equality," and below that it says, "'nuff said." Ironically, there is plenty more to be said about the implication of this popular false concept. The reason this argument for equality fails is because it attempts to equate human properties that are not equivalent. One's race or ethnicity is not equivalent to one's sexuality, which is not equivalent to one's belief or lack of belief in God. Therefore, to mix all these properties together and phrase it in this manner is wholly deceptive. Now, are we all human? Absolutely. Do we all have skeletons? Absolutely. However, immorality is not equivalent to morality, which is our focus here. Morality is weighed by the contents of our hearts and is manifested in our thoughts, speech, and actions, not in our skeletons. So if homosexuality is immoral, it is not equivalent to sexual morality—i.e., God's parameters for sex, which is exclusively between one man and one woman within the permanent bond of marriage. Understanding this, "everyone is equal," simply fails to prove that homosexuality is not sinful.

**6. "You should just love everyone and treat everyone with kindness."**
***Logical Fallacy Committed:*** *Irrelevant Conclusion Fallacy*—reaching a conclusion that is irrelevant to the argument.

The claim that we should love everyone and treat everyone with kindness is absolutely true. However, there is a hidden implication here that I must point out, which is: to question or oppose homosexuality is to be unkind and hateful. This implication is plainly false. We can question or oppose homosexuality and still treat "homosexuals" with love and kindness. It happens all the time. In fact, this is the obligation of every Christian because Jesus Christ Himself operated in this fashion. Jesus even showed love and kindness to Judas *even as he betrayed Him*. If the Bible says we are to even love our enemies, there is no excuse for us to not treat everyone with love and kindness. "Homosexuals" are not our enemies, so obviously we are obligated to treat them with love and kindness as well. This is what I practice, and this is what the Christians I know practice. I've even had debates with "homosexuals" who sharply disagreed with me, but in the end they thanked me for offering a logical respectful argument. So something is clearly amiss, and we need to determine what treating someone with love and kindness actually entails. Does it mean remaining silent and withholding the truth in order to spare someone's feelings? Does it mean ignoring or condoning someone's sinful behavior? Does it mean allowing someone to drift further and further away from God as they damage themselves and others? No, no, and no. To truly love someone is to tell them the truth; to help them abstain from sin and to save them, not to ignore or condone their sinful behavior.

So in the discussion of morality and homosexuality, to claim "You should just love everyone and treat everyone with kindness," is not a conclusion to be reached or evidence to support answering "no" to the question at hand. In fact, even though it's something true Christians already practice, it is entirely irrelevant to our topic. The reason we are determining the moral status of homosexuality is *because* we love and care about "homosexuals." Thus, this argument also fails to prove homosexuality is not sinful.

**7. "There's nothing wrong with people who are in love being together."**
*Logical Fallacy Committed: Moralistic Fallacy—*"X ought to be right. Therefore X is right."

This is a bold truth claim. Whenever presented with a truth claim, you should immediately ask yourself, "Is that actually true?" So in this instance, is there *truly* nothing wrong with people who are in love being together? It's one thing to make a truth claim; it's another thing entirely to *prove* a truth claim with concrete evidence. So where is the concrete evidence for this truth claim? I've yet to be provided with any. If the presence of love is the qualifier for an acceptable moral relationship, then what is that principle based on? It appears to me that a great majority of people desire this to be true, and so they decide, whether consciously or unconsciously, that it is indeed true. The truth, however, is this truth claim is entirely irrational—it's based on feelings and opinions instead of facts and reason—and on top of that it commits a logical fallacy.

There is also more to this truth claim than those who present it are aware of. If they are attempting to use love to justify the morality of homosexuality, then what about "homosexual" couples who are not in love? Are they not immoral by default because of the absence of love in their sexual relationships? Practicing "homosexuals" who are single and simply desire the freedom to have unrestricted sexual relationships make up a significant portion of the "homosexual" community. Based on this truth claim they fall outside of the category of a "loving couple" and therefore cannot also be considered moral.

It's fascinating listening to the range of responses to this line of questioning. I had a discussion with a Christian coworker who was a proponent of homosexuality. He explained that he simply refused to believe God would condemn such nice and wonderful people simply because of their "sexual orientation." In the beginning of our conversation, the moral line he'd drawn included "homosexual" practice in its entirety. It was interesting, however, that he began to shift his own moral line as we examined the clear difference between monogamous "homosexual" couples and single promiscuous "homosexuals." He altered his stance by quickly declaring the latter was definitely wrong. Who's to say in time he won't alter his stance again and say homosexuality in its entirety is wrong?

Further, why stop at "homosexual" relationships? There are many other relationship types that seek justification based on their "love." Those would also have to be accepted based on the ambiguous assertion that there's nothing wrong with people in love being together. A couple of years ago I participated in a friendly online debate on homosexuality, and a proponent of homosexuality made this truth claim, implying that as long as two people are in love, there's nothing wrong with it. I then presented a scenario with three different couples for her consideration: a man and a young girl, a man and his sister, and a man and his dog.

"Is nothing wrong with these relationships if they are truly in love?" I asked. Unfortunately, at that point someone I didn't know joined the debate and was enraged by my question.

"How dare you compare those relationships to gay couples!" she posted, and then proceeded to call me all sorts of foul names. This young lady totally missed the point of my question and steered a healthy debate way off track. The point is that if love is all that's necessary to justify a sexual relationship, then the line cannot simply be drawn at "homosexual" couples. This young lady argued the couples I'd used in my scenario were preposterous and insinuated that they were obviously immoral. She would be surprised to learn, however, that under the umbrella of the Sexual Freedom Movement along with "gay rights," there is also a movement to normalize these exact relationships and others of an even more bizarre nature. They attempt to justify this by using the same logically fallacious claim that there's nothing wrong with people in love being together. There is actually an organization called NAMBLA (North American Man/Boy Love Association). According to their website: NAMBLA's goal is to end the extreme oppression of men and boys in mutually consensual relationships by:

- building understanding and support for such relationships;
- educating the general public on the benevolent nature of man/boy love;
- cooperating with lesbian, gay, feminist, and other liberation movements; supporting the liberation of persons of all ages from sexual prejudice and oppression.[17]

An Australian judge named Garry Neilson was suspended from presiding over criminal cases because he claimed that incest was only a criminal act because of the abnormalities in the resulting offspring. He said, "But even that falls away to an extent [because] there is such ease of contraception and readily access to abortion."[18] I saw an article that showed a young man marrying his dog. They had an outdoor ceremony, the dog wore a veil, and after the vows were exchanged (I'm not certain how the dog managed this part), the man kneeled down and kissed the dog in the mouth. So what was deemed totally outlandish by an angry, yet passionate advocate only a couple years ago is now not only being promoted in this push for "sexual freedom," but these relationships actual exist and are being justified by "love."

It doesn't end there. I thought I'd heard it all, but I was terribly wrong. Have you ever heard the term "throuple"? The first time I heard it I was completely baffled and had to look it up to see what it meant. It turns out that a "throuple" is a relationship with three members of the same sex. Three "lesbian" women have deemed themselves the first "throuple" and had a mock wedding ceremony to consummate their love: "Doll, Kitten, and Brynn Young exchanged vows in a commitment ceremony last August, with all three brides wearing white and traditional wedding veils."[19] This was followed by a male "throuple" in Taiwan who became an internet sensation after they got "married," arguing there is nothing wrong with their union because "love is love." Art, one of the three grooms, posted, "Love occurs unconditionally and is not limited to only two people. Love brings peace to the world."[20]

As if that wasn't enough, there is something called a "quartet." This is a relationship with four individuals (apparently some quartets include two males and two females) who are all in love with one another and wish to consummate their love through marriage as well.

Stranger yet, I read an incredibly unsettling article about a girl and her biological father who are in love and have aspirations of getting "married."[21]

Obviously, we must ask ourselves, is anything wrong with these people who love each other being together? To answer "no" is to be dishonest. If you say, "Yes, there's definitely something wrong with those relationships," where do you draw the line that shouldn't be crossed? If you draw the line at "homosexual" couples and say they are acceptable, but nothing beyond that, someone else might say the line should be drawn at "throuples" or "quartets", while still another would argue the line should be drawn at consensual incest and pedophilia. So who has the power and authority to draw the official line between sexually immoral relationships and sexually moral relationships? You? If so, why is the line you draw more valid than the line someone else draws? Who is right? The government? Surely we can't believe something becomes moral simply because the government writes it into law. Slavery was once lawful, that didn't make slavery moral. So how can we set a new precedent to rationalize homosexuality based on love but nothing beyond that? What's more, who's to say the line you draw today is the same line you'll draw tomorrow? These are the questions one must answer when attempting to redefine the parameters of love and sexually moral relationships. If we are honest with ourselves, we will realize none of us have the power to dictate the morality of any sexual relationship because none of us are perfect, none of us have unlimited knowledge, nor did any of us create mankind, marriage, or sex. None of us are identified as love itself. Therefore, none of us are capable of redefining the nature and purpose of these creations.

Further, it must be pointed out that because someone claims to love someone that doesn't mean it is truly love. Sure, they can believe it and feel it with the whole of their being and say, "Who are you to tell me I don't love my partner?" The answer is, "I'm nobody. I know I did not set the parameters for love, because I'm terribly incapable to do so like every other person on the planet." The truth is God is the only Being in existence qualified to set the parameters for love because He is love. Love is a great deal more than a series of emotions, and sexual urges, which result from attraction and compatibility. Love by God's definition is never sinful; it is never immoral. Therefore, if anyone's concept of love leads to sin, then it is not love; it is lust, and lust is sinful.

In light of these facts, the claim, "There's nothing wrong with people who are in love being together" is plainly false. After all, people attempt to justify adulterous relationships by using love as an excuse, but there's obviously something wrong with married individuals having extra-marital affairs. Adultery is sinful regardless if the adulterers are in love or not. So it is clear that evoking love does absolutely nothing to absolve the sinfulness of sexually immoral relationships. Consequently, this argument clearly fails to prove that homosexuality is not sinful.

In the next chapter we will continue our thorough examination of the final three arguments that attempt to prove homosexuality is not sinful.

# 3

# Is Homosexuality Sinful?
# The "No" Position (II)

**8. "They're Born That Way."**
***Logical Fallacies Committed:*** *False Cause*—presuming a
relationship between two things means one caused the other.
*Appeal to Nature*—the assertion that because something is
"natural" it is justified or good.

Before examining this truth claim, I want to make something clear. There is a fierce ongoing debate between those
who insist that "homosexuals" are born that way and those
who insist "homosexuals" choose to be that way. I call this
the "born vs. choice debate," and I believe it is utterly fruitless. In fact, after reading a lengthy debate online that went
nowhere and helped no one, I hoped to quell the argument by
focusing on what is far more important than the cause of the
"homosexual" disposition. I posted a message online asserting
the "born vs. choice debate" is irrelevant because the former
cannot be proven, and the latter does not hold true in all cases.

Not everyone who experiences SSA does so as a matter of choice—particularly those who suffered sexual molestation/ abuse as a child and struggle with homosexuality as a direct result. That clearly wasn't a choice but a result of a tragic experience. Therefore, we should all focus on what is truly important, which is that regardless if we identify as "gay" or "straight," it is not how we are born that matters. It's how we live, if we love God more than anything and anyone else, and where we'll spend eternity that truly matters. Yet, as I previously referenced, although my post was entirely positive, the majority of the responses I received were not only negative, they were hostile. What's more, most of those who took issue with my post decided to disregard the main point, which again was positive. Instead, they poured all of their energy into continuing the endless "born vs. choice debate," which is totally irrelevant here because neither position determines the moral status of homosexuality. Even if it was universally accepted that all "homosexuals" were born that way, that wouldn't prove homosexuality is not sinful. Consequently, I find it a waste of time, energy, and opportunity to try to "win" this never-ending argument, and I highly recommend you don't fall into this trap.

That being said, "They're born that way," is a truth claim that I've heard so often that instead of responding with guess-work or opinion, I opted to follow my own protocol and immediately ask, "Is this truth claim actually true?" I then diligently sought out the factual evidence to draw the proper conclusion. What follows is not ammunition to be used to try to win this argument, but is merely the collection of facts I uncovered. I believe the truth will benefit everyone and elim-inate the confusion and controversy surrounding this "born vs. choice debate." Perhaps then we can finally put it to rest and focus on what matters most.

Now, let's address the first logical fallacy this argument commits, which is the *False Cause* fallacy. It is illogical to assume that because an individual identifies as a "homosexual" that the cause was the way they were born. Still, many people wholly believe that connection is valid. To support this belief I've often heard: "Nobody would ever choose to be gay. Nobody would choose to be discriminated against and oppressed by society." With the concept of choice eliminated, it is then assumed that the sole alternative is that those who identify as "homosexuals" were born with an unavoidable "homosexual" disposition. To add further weight to this claim, many people argue that they know someone who showed signs of being "gay" from an early age, which, in their minds, qualifies as proof of people being born "homosexual." I found several things interesting about this argument.

a) Many believe in the existence of the fabled "gay gene," but the fact is there is no credible scientific evidence to prove people are born "homosexual." Although the search for this "gay gene" has continued for years, it has never been discovered because it does not exist. Of course, there are those who looked up some studies on the internet and offer the results of those studies as "scientific proof" that people are born "homosexual." However, as I'm sure you're well aware, you can find anything on the internet—that doesn't mean that it is true or accurate. Those who fully research the issue using credible references from credible scientists discover why those studies are inaccurate and have thus been universally rejected. This alone is enough evidence to dismiss the notion that people are born "homosexual," but there's far more to consider.

b) Genetic traits (characteristics that people are born with) cannot be reversed at will. Freckles, dimples, and colorblindness are examples of genetic traits. Obviously, a person cannot merely decide they will no longer have freckles, or dimples, or be colorblind.

These characteristics are written into their genetic code. This is important to understand, because in regards to homosexuality, not only do "ex-gays" exist, but they exist in vast numbers. Dr. Neil Whitehead authored the book *My Genes Made Me Do It,* which compiles more than twenty years of research on homosexuality. The research shows:

> *...The huge amount of change in sexual orientation is one of the clearest evidences that homosexuality is not hard-wired by genes or anything in the biological environment . . . Numbers of people who have changed towards exclusive OSA are greater than current numbers of bisexuals and exclusive SSA people combined. In other words, Ex-gays outnumber actual gays.*[22]

If there was indeed a "gay gene," this reversal from SSA to exclusive OSA would be impossible. Yet there are countless individuals who identified as "homosexual" for years, some for several decades, but have since abandoned homosexuality and never returned. Many of them are now happily married with children. This serves as proof that homosexuality is not genetic.

c) If people were truly born gay, if the "homosexual" disposition was actually a product of genetics, then we would see proof of that in identical twins. If people were born "homosexual", then whenever one identical twin is "homosexual", the other twin would also be "homosexual" *every time*. According to Dr. Whitehead: "Identical twins have the same genes or DNA. They are nurtured in equal prenatal conditions. If homosexuality is caused by genetics or prenatal conditions and one twin is gay, the co-twin should also be gay. Because they have identical DNA, it ought to be one hundred percent." However, the studies reveal something else. "If an identical twin has same-sex attraction the chances the co-twin has it are only about eleven percent for men and fourteen perfect for women." Because identical twins are always genetically identical, homosexuality cannot be genetically dictated. "No-one is born gay," Dr. Whitehead declares. "The predominant things that create homosexuality in one identical twin and not in the other have to be post-birth factors."[22]

d) People assume there are only two possible explanations for a person's "homosexual" disposition—they're either born "gay" or they chose to be "gay." In their minds, if it's not one it must be the other. In truth the "homosexual" disposition is a consequence of a wide number of factors that take place between the time of birth and the time one chooses to identify as "homosexual." The list of causes for homosexuality include: a conscious decision; experimentation; confusion; a dysfunctional home environment; suffering and/or witnessing abuse; emotional neglect; physical neglect; exposure to pornography or sexual situations; being raised by a single parent; emotional brokenness with one or both parents, siblings, or peers; labeling; bullying; media influence; rebellion (natural and/or spiritual); lust; addictions; or any combination of these. This is not even an exhaustive list. The fact is everyone who identifies as "homosexual" can't be put into the same box. There are multiple factors at work regarding the cause of one's "homosexual" disposition that are often ignored, undetermined, or misunderstood, but that in no way proves the cause is birth.

e) Effeminate characteristics in young males and masculine characteristics in young females do not always result in a "homosexual" disposition. I've had many great discussions about individuals who showed signs of being "homosexual" from various young ages. "Isn't that proof they were born gay?" people often ask. Not necessarily. For over a decade I've had the pleasure of working with children of various ages, and I've witnessed young boys who acted more like girls and young girls who acted more like boys. In today's society people would immediately start labeling these children as "gay" or "transgender," as if there's no possible alternative, but there *is* a possible alternative: they're neither "gay" nor "transgender." Shocking isn't it? While growing up, I had a group of friends I played with all the time. One of the boys in the group was different from the others. He was sensitive and often preferred playing with the girls instead of us boys. While we were all outside horsing around or playing with LEGOS or He-Man figures (remember those?), he wanted to play Barbie with the girls. This struck everyone as odd, but no one denied him. At times he was even content to play with Barbie dolls by himself while all the other kids played together. Again, many people today would have immediately labeled him as "gay" and treated him as though he were a "homosexual" from that moment on. This would have been an error because he is not "gay." He has never been confused about his sexuality, and thirty years later, he is currently in a long-term relationship with his girlfriend. So we cannot support the claim that people are born "gay" by relying on the fact that some kids act certain ways or play with certain toys. They are kids. Everyone who has kids of their own or has worked with kids for a number of years can attest that the way children act when they are young does not inevitably endure for the rest of their lives.

f) All "homosexuals" don't believe they were born gay. Every person I know who identifies as "homosexual," and was kind enough to share their stories with me, have told me plainly they were not born that way. Likewise, my brother, who has more "homosexual" friends than I do, was curious about this issue and asked all of them if they believed they were born "gay." Every single one of them said that they were not. There was a video going around entitled "Undercover Video of Gays Admitting they are not 'Born that way,'" which is a compilation of individuals in the "LGBT" community who detail what led to their "homosexual" identification. Being born that way was not anyone's story. One would think that if there were truth to the claim that the "homosexual" disposition is a direct result of birth, then one hundred percent of "homosexuals" would agree on this. They don't. Further, it's important to understand what "They choose to be that way," actually means. It does not suggest that people choose to experience SSA. It does, however, mean practicing "homosexuals" choose how they identify themselves, and they choose to act on their sexual attractions. In other words, practicing "homosexuals" chose to "come out" as a "homosexual" and they chose to practice homosexuality. Once again, not everyone who experiences SSA chooses to identify as "gay" or act on those attractions. These are all choices, and everyone is held accountable for their choices. With that said, I know this remains a highly sensitive matter and that some "homosexuals" adamantly insist they were born "gay," and that is fine. I do my best to respect everyone's right to believe whatever they wish. Still, it is important to remember our goal here is to set our feelings and opinions aside and simply consider the facts so we can move past this issue to what's more important.

Now let's address the second logical fallacy committed by those who claim "they're born that way." To commit the *Appeal to Nature* fallacy is to disregard the fact that because something is "natural" that does not make it moral. The claim "they're born that way" suggests "homosexuals" can't help but to indulge in homosexuality. If they were born that way, then it is natural, and if it is natural, then it is moral. This is obviously fallacious reasoning because this doesn't apply to any other area in life. There are people who seem to have a natural propensity for violent behavior. Does that mean for them it's moral to act on those impulses and commit violent acts? Of course not. More to the point, I will reiterate I am a male with an attraction to females I don't think is normal. I am *insanely* attracted to females. So could I use the argument that because I was born this way, it is normal for me to act on my heightened attraction to females by having promiscuous sex and call that moral behavior? Absolutely not. I know pre-marital sex is immoral behavior, which is why I fight daily to keep my sexual impulses under control so I do not behave immorally. Sometimes, I literally have to put cartoons on and watch some Tom & Jerry to clear my mind of sexual thoughts in order to maintain my purity. So clearly this idea that what is natural is moral is plainly false. Camille Paglia, who identifies as both a "lesbian" and a pagan, unashamedly tells the truth about homosexuality despite the backlash she receives from her "LGBT" peers. Camille said:

> *Homosexuality is not "normal." On the contrary, it is a challenge to the norm . . . Nature exists, whether academics like it or not. And in nature, procreation is the single relentless*

*rule. That is the norm. Our sexual bodies were designed for reproduction. Penis fits vagina; no fancy linguistic game playing can change that biological fact.*[23]

S. Michael Craven, author of *Uncompromised Faith: Overcoming Our Culturalized Christianity,* confirms this fact:

*We are born biologically male or female and as such we are sexually dissimilar, but in complementary ways. The male/female sexual union works, in other words. This is true of every species on earth. Every living organism has a particular way of reproducing and rearing offspring; its anatomy is biologically designed to support that way. If one believes we are products of an evolutionary process, then "homosexual" acts are a deviation from the procreative design and homosexuality is therefore a genetic defect, because it fails to propagate the species. If one holds to the belief that we are created, then it defies the design and intent of the Creator. Either way homosexuality violates the given design.*[24]

What we've learned here is the claim "they're born that way" simply can't be proven because it is false. Even if it were true, that still wouldn't prove that homosexuality is not sinful. This brings us right back to our original inquiry—*is homosexuality sinful?* "They're born that way" fails to answer that question. We must move past this point and recognize as free moral agents we are all held morally accountable for the decisions we make. According to the Bible we are *all* born into sin. Every one of us has a sinful nature that we must overcome in order to live a moral, Godly lifestyle. Therefore, *none of us* can use the argument "I was born that way" as an excuse to live a sinful lifestyle.

**9. "Jesus never spoke against homosexuality."**
*Logical Fallacy Committed: Confirmation Bias*—relying on evidence that confirms one's preconceived belief while ignoring and/or rejecting all evidence contrary to that belief.

Those who commit this logical fallacy are actually saying: "I've already decided what I believe, and I'll continue to believe it regardless if it's actually true or not." This is a dangerous mindset, as it ignores all facts and reason contrary to one's erroneous belief. It is essentially self-deception by denial. Let us examine why this argument about Jesus falls into this category and how it fails to legitimize homosexuality. Can anyone actually confirm Jesus never specifically spoke against homosexuality? No. None of us were there to hear every word that Jesus ever spoke, and the Bible certainly didn't record His every word either. This alone proves that this bold assertion is conjecture, not fact.

Nevertheless, let's assume that this assertion is true. Does it then mean whatever Jesus did not speak about is automatically acceptable or moral? Obviously not. One could argue Jesus never singled out and condemned rape or bestiality either, yet those acts are clearly sinful. Why then, should homosexuality be an exception? Further, one could easily counter this biased assertion by pointing out the obvious fact that Jesus never spoke *for* homosexuality. This is factual for two reasons: everything Jesus said in the Bible regarding sexually morality excludes homosexuality, and it is impossible for Jesus to contradict himself, thus anything he said outside of the biblical record would not possibly be in favor of homosexuality. Let's continue by examining what Jesus actually did say, instead of assuming what He didn't say. First, it's important to establish that homosexuality is a modern word, so it is unfair to assume Jesus would use a term that is familiar to us but unfamiliar to the ancient world. Thus the real question is whether or not Jesus addressed what we know today as homosexuality in the language that they actually used at that time. The answer is *yes*. Jesus spoke against homosexuality both directly and indirectly. In the infamous Sermon on the Mount, Jesus specifically condemned sexual immorality:

> What comes out of a man is what makes him "unclean." For from within, out of men's hearts, come evil thoughts, *sexual immorality*, theft, murder, adultery, greed, malice, deceit, lewdness, envy, slander, arrogance and folly. All these evils come from inside and make a man "unclean" (Mark 7:20–23).

So what exactly is sexual immorality? Sexual immorality is the English translation of the original Greek term *porneia*, which is the term that Jesus used in the aforementioned Scripture. *Porneia*, when defined specifically, denotes every form of illicit sexual intercourse, which points directly to the sexually condemned acts identified in the book of Leviticus: adultery, fornication, homosexuality, incest, and bestiality. So in declaring that sexual immorality is evil and makes a man unclean, Jesus specifically condemned homosexuality and all other premarital and extramarital sexual activities as evil. Further, there was no ambiguity to Jesus' message; that which Jesus condemned was well understood by His audience.

Notice that not only does homosexuality fall into the category of sexual immorality, which Jesus clearly identified as evil, but lewdness is also identified as evil. Lewd means to be obscene and sexually unchaste, and yet lewdness is a fundamental component of the "homosexual" culture. It is therefore quite clear that Jesus did indeed reference homosexuality, and He condemned it. Now you might ask why

Jesus didn't *specifically* single out homosexuality when condemning sexual immorality. Well, if you're familiar with the Bible, you are well aware in the Old Testament God gave the Law to Moses, who delivered it to the Israelites, and the Law clearly forbade "homosexual" activity. If Jesus never specifically singled out homosexuality, it wasn't because He approved of it, but because condemning it would have been redundant. For generations the Israelites meticulously followed the Law or paid the penalty for violating it, and the Jews of Jesus' day still followed the Mosaic Law and knew it intimately. They clearly understood "homosexual" activity was expressly forbidden. The Israelites were selected by God to be His holy people and a shining example to the rest of the world. Consequently, their penalty for violating God's law by committing "homosexual" acts was extreme—they were to be put to death. It is easy to see why homosexuality was not prevalent in the Jewish community when Jesus walked the earth. Considering this, it would have been odd for Jesus to single out homosexuality after reaffirming that all sexual immorality is sinful.

Now, if the Law had changed, Jesus would have made that distinction just as He did in other areas. For example, before Christ it was necessary to commit the physical act to be guilty of adultery. After Christ, He made it quite clear that even looking on a woman with lust in one's heart makes a man guilty of adultery. Therefore, if God were to change His mind and decide homosexuality was no longer detestable or an abomination to Him (which is impossible because God's Moral Law never changes), Jesus would have made that perfectly clear. Obviously, He did not make such an amendment to the previous commands forbidding homosexuality.

Now let's look at how Jesus indirectly condemned homosexuality as sinful. Jesus reaffirmed God's design for marriage by quoting God's words recorded in the book of Genesis.

> "Haven't you read," He replied, "that at the beginning the Creator 'made them male and female,' and said, 'For this reason a man will leave his father and mother and be united to his wife, and the two will become one flesh'? So they are no longer two, but one. Therefore what God has joined together, let man not separate (Matthew 19:4–6).

This reaffirmation not only explicitly details God's design for marriage and emphasizes the permanence of the union; it also reaffirms the parameters and purpose for sex. Notice who does the joining. God joins man and woman together in marriage. They don't join themselves. The "becoming one flesh," or the sexual union between husband and wife, is a sacred symbolic act. It reflects and commemorates the union God created and it follows His design for procreation and family. Thus to remove God, and remove His marriage from a sexual relationship and claim whatever results is moral, is clearly false, as it is a total distortion of God's perfect design.

Although I've already provided enough evidence to easily dismiss this argument, there's even more to consider. If Jesus was sent to the Jews to whom He condemned all sexual immorality, then what about the Gentiles (non-Jewish people)? Who was sent to speak to them? The Apostle Paul was selected for this task. Who handpicked the Apostle Paul to carry the gospel to the Gentiles? Jesus did. Homosexuality was as prevalent among the Gentiles then as it is today, even though the concept of a "homosexual orientation" was foreign. As a result Paul was tasked with tackling this issue head on. He was responsible for teaching the Gentiles that God strictly forbade homosexuality and every other version of sexual immorality. The Gentiles never had this law before like the Jews did, and so it was essential that this command was drilled into their minds. Given that Jesus personally selected Paul to carry the gospel to the Gentiles, what Paul said was an extension of Jesus' ministry; so the truth of this message can absolutely be attributed to Christ.

When asserting what Jesus said and did not say, it's also important to remember Jesus and God are one. Thus, we cannot exclude Jesus from anything that God has said, and God specifically condemned homosexuality. Additionally, Jesus is the Word, the Word (or Bible) condemns homosexuality; therefore, Jesus condemns homosexuality.

The evidence is abundantly clear, and the assertion that "Jesus never spoke against homosexuality," is plainly false. It is impossible to justify homosexuality (or "gay marriage") by making this false claim. Particularly when considering the whole of Scripture, which condemns homosexuality and sets the parameters for sexual morality and marriage. Anyone who attempts to use the Bible and/or Jesus Christ as a means to justify homosexuality will fail every time because neither the Bible nor Jesus ever justifies homosexuality. Ultimately, this argument has been proven irrational, illogical, and untrue, and thus it utterly fails to legitimize homosexuality in any way.

**10. "The Scriptures against homosexuality have been misinterpreted/mistranslated."**
*Fallacy:* a false notion or belief

Where the previous nine assertions committed at least one logical fallacy (an error in reasoning), this one is simply a fallacy. Once again, we must immediately question this bold truth claim. Some people actually take this accusation even further, claiming the entire Bible has been mistranslated, or that it can be interpreted in so many ways that it's impossible to use it as a valid source of authority. The truth, however, is the Bible is the most authentic historical document known to man. In fact, no other historical document even comes close to the authenticity of the Bible. If you've done any credible research on the Bible, you know this is not conjecture; this is fact. The Bible is utterly unique, it is inerrant, and the only explanation for the Bible surviving the ages and being proven accurate and consistent is that God was directly involved in its inception, distribution, and preservation. What's interesting is the common challenges against the Bible as an accurate and authoritative source are often made by individuals who have not even read the Bible or done any credible research on the Bible. They regurgitate what they've heard *about* the Bible or what they've read on the internet. So audacious claims like "The Bible is full of contradictions," "The Bible was written by men," (whatever that's supposed to mean), and "The Bible has been rewritten so many times it's full of errors," are easily dismissible with proper examination. What's more, today we have the benefit of technology, so any one of us can look up the original languages of the Bible, study the translation, and understand the nuances of the original languages to prove the Bible we have today was accurately translated. We can be quite confident the Bible is a credible source of authority.

This claim that the Scriptures on homosexuality have been misinterpreted or mistranslated is a counterattack of sorts. It is no mystery that the Bible condemns "homosexual" behavior, and consequently it has long been the majority position that homosexuality is sinful. Many advocates have reasoned if the Bible is wrong, then this whole position falls apart, which is actually a valid inference. This begs the question: is the Bible wrong about homosexuality? Were the Scriptures concerning homosexuality translated accurately? Unfortunately, many of those who challenge Scripture don't care to find out because they *want* to Bible to be wrong. This is where rational thought is replaced with irrational thought. Their illogical reasoning goes like this:

1.  I'm a "homosexual" (or people I know and love are "homosexuals").

2. The Bible says homosexuality is sinful.
3. I don't want homosexuality to be sinful.
4. Therefore, I'll either refuse to believe in the Bible, or I'll believe the Bible wasn't translated accurately.
5. Then I will be justified in my "homosexual" lifestyle (or the people I know and love will be justified in their "homosexual" lifestyle).

This line of reasoning obviously fails to disprove the Bible's account of homosexuality. The desire for something to be a certain way doesn't magically make it that way. We must rely on what is factual, not on what we wish was factual.

Others take a more aggressive approach and actually seek to discredit every Scripture in the Bible that mentions homosexuality. We'll take a look at these Scriptures, the objections against them, and determine if these Scriptures should be adhered to or disregarded. In Genesis 19 we find the infamous story of Sodom and Gomorrah. The citizens of these two ancient cities were incredibly immoral. When two angels visited the city of Sodom, the men there actually desired to rape them. Their sexual perversion was so offensive to God that He destroyed those two cities by raining burning sulfur upon them. Leviticus 18:22 records the words of God himself, which Moses passed on to the Israelites: "Do not lie with a man as one lies with a woman; that is detestable." This command is reiterated in Leviticus 20:13, which says, "If a man lies with a man as one lies with a woman, both of them have done what is detestable." The commands forbidding all "homosexual" activity continue in the New Testament, beginning with the most descriptive prohibition of homosexuality in the Bible. In Romans 1:24–28 the Apostle Paul says:

> Therefore God gave them over in the sinful desires of their hearts to sexual impurity for the degrading of their bodies with one another.

> They exchanged the truth of God for a lie, and worshiped and served created things rather than the Creator—who is forever praised. Amen. Because of this, God gave them over to shameful lusts. Even their women exchanged natural relations for unnatural ones. In the same way the men also abandoned natural relations with women and were inflamed with lust for one another. Men committed indecent acts with other men, and received in themselves the due penalty for their perversion. Furthermore, since they did not think it worthwhile to retain the knowledge of God, he gave them over to a depraved mind, to do what ought not to be done.

Following this, in 1 Corinthians 6:9–10 the Apostle Paul says:

> Do you not know that the wicked will not inherit the kingdom of God? Do not be deceived: Neither the sexually immoral nor idolaters nor adulterers nor male prostitutes nor homosexual offenders nor thieves nor the greedy nor drunkards nor slanderers nor swindlers will inherit the kingdom of God.

Finally, in 1 Timothy 1:9–10 Paul says again:

> We also know that the law is made not for the righteous but for lawbreakers and rebels, the ungodly and sinful, the unholy and irreligious, for those who kill their fathers or mothers, for murderers, for the sexually immoral, for those practicing homosexuality, for slave traders

and liars and perjurers—and for whatever else
is contrary to the sound doctrine (NIV 2010).

So as we've seen, the Bible expressly forbids all "homosexual" practice in six specific Scriptures—three in the Old
Testament and three in the New Testament. It's important to
point out that the repetition of a biblical command is a strong
indication that the command is *extremely* important.

Although these six Scriptures individually and collectively make God's position on homosexuality perfectly and
abundantly clear, you would be amazed at the ways people
have challenged the validity of these Scriptures in an effort
to rationalize homosexuality. Let's look at these challenges
one by one. Proponents of homosexuality have posited in
Genesis 19 the crime for which the cities of Sodom and
Gomorrah were destroyed was not homosexuality but a lack
of hospitality. In other words, when the two angels came
to the city of Sodom, the people did not revere them and
treat them with hospitality, and that was the offense that
resulted in the cities being destroyed. This, in itself, is an
erroneous attempt to disregard this Scripture for several reasons. First of all, the angels weren't in Gomorrah when they
suffered this "lack of hospitality," so if that was truly the
crime, it would have been unfair to destroy Gomorrah as well.
Secondly, the Bible (which again, has gone unread by most
of those who like to challenge what it says,) proves this accusation completely false. In Jude 7 we find the exact reason
Sodom and Gomorrah were destroyed, and it had absolutely
nothing to do with hospitality. "In a similar way, Sodom
and Gomorrah and the surrounding towns gave themselves
up to sexual immorality and perversion. They serve as an
example of those who suffer the punishment of eternal fire."
Furthermore, God decided to destroy those cities *before* even
sending the angels to visit Lot. In Genesis 18:20–21 God
said, "The outcry against Sodom and Gomorrah is so great

and their sin so grievous that I will go down and see if what they have done is as bad as the outcry that has reached me." Again, this was *before* the men of Sodom attempted to rape the angels, which proves that hospitality was never in question. Now, God knows all things, so He knew the people of Sodom would try to rape His angels, and yet He sent them anyway. Why? It was to prove to Lot and Abraham that there were indeed no righteous people there to warrant sparing the two cities. The people were entirely unrighteous because they were sexually immoral and perverse and thus ripe for destruction. We can therefore completely dismiss this ludicrous assertion that the reason Sodom and Gomorrah were destroyed had to do with anything other than sexual perversion, specifically homosexuality.

Attempts to dismiss Leviticus 18:22 and 20:13, which specifically condemn homosexuality, usually fall into one of two categories:

1. "These Scriptures aren't referring to homosexuality."
2. "Leviticus doesn't apply to Christians today."

Let's examine these by looking at some real-life arguments. We'll begin with the first category. "Tom," a young man I know, is a professing Christian and an "out and proud" "homosexual." He told me that homosexuality isn't a sin and was more than willing to discuss how he reached that conclusion. What was the basis of his argument? His "research" and discussions with professors at his Christian college led him to believe these Scriptures don't refer to homosexuality; they refer to rape. According to him, it was a common practice for men to rape their defeated enemies in times of war and this was what God commanded the Israelites to abstain from. I showed him how this theory immediately fails. If "Do not lie with a man as one lies with a woman" is indeed a reference to rape, then it would actually be condoning the rape of women! The Scripture would essentially read, "Do not rape a man as one rapes a woman." This is obviously absurd. Further, Moses, the author of Leviticus, condemns rape repeatedly in his other writings and the word rape is actually used. When the word rape is not used but described instead, the description of the deplorable act is nothing like what we read in these two Leviticus Scriptures. For example, when Moses described rape in Genesis 34:2 he said, "he took her and violated her." The difference is obvious and it is clearly impossible that the Leviticus Scriptures referred to anything other than homosexuality. Tom, who was so convinced these Scriptures were about rape and was so excited to use this as a means to rationalize homosexuality, suddenly had no rebuttal. He merely said that he would respond after "praying about it." That response never came, which speaks volumes, but I pray one day it does and that I am able to help him.

The second category involves the attempt to dismiss the entire book of Leviticus. Those who take this route base their argument on the fact that Leviticus is filled with a host of other commands that are disregarded by Christians today. Time and time again I've heard these sorts of arguments, even from professing Christians. An advocate friend of mine said, "The Bible does not clearly state that homosexuality is wrong. Leviticus is just a book of laws that were applicable to that culture and that time period. Leviticus also says that we can't eat pork or shrimp or get tattoos so we can't just pick out homosexuality and excuse the rest of these things." Another professing Christian I know argued, "How do you choose that homosexuality is sinful from the Bible as law, but continue to shave your face, eat meat, wear polyester, and not stone adulterers to death?" If you've ever had a debate about homosexuality, I'm sure you've heard similar arguments against the book of Leviticus. Are these good and valid arguments? No they aren't. The errors made by those who try to dismiss God's commands against homosexuality by listing

commands that don't apply to Christians are ignoring three fundamental principles in their interpretation of Scripture.
1. The Bible contains the *Ceremonial Law* and the *Moral Law*. It is absolutely critical to understand the content and nature of each. The Ceremonial Law includes commands the Israelites were obligated to follow in order to be purified before Christ came. These included sacrifices and rituals, and all of those previously mentioned traditions that people love to bring up in an attempt to rationalize homosexuality. By contrast, the Moral Law includes God's commands that apply to *all* mankind, not only the ancient Israelites. The Ceremonial Law began with Moses and expired with Jesus Christ. The Moral Law began with God and never expires. All commandments concerning sexual immorality are part of God's Moral Law. Thus, one cannot use an obsolete command from the Ceremonial Law, which does not apply to *anyone* today, as grounds of dismissing any part of the Moral Law, which applies to *everyone* today and is eternal. This principle also applies to the popular argument comparing "detestable" behaviors: "Yes God said homosexuality was detestable in Leviticus, but God said a lot of other things were detestable that we practice today so this proves homosexuality is acceptable." This argument fails on two accounts. First, against the backdrop of the aforementioned distinction between the Moral and Ceremonial Laws, it is clear what was detestable for the Israelites pre-Christ, but is now acceptable for Christians today, is in no way linked to what was detestable for everyone pre-Christ, and is still detestable for everyone post-Christ. In other words, shaving one's face cannot be linked to homosexuality. Second, the Bible's consistent condemnation of homosexuality is confirmed by

the fact that the New Testament reaffirms the sinfulness of homosexuality. We cannot simply discount
Old Testament Scripture and think that gives us
license to approve of and/or indulge in homosexuality, especially when the New Testament Scriptures
are in harmony with the Old Testament in forbidding
"homosexual" practice. It's amazing how many times
I've been in debates where people attack all the Old
Testament Scriptures but completely ignore the New
Testament. I've also been in debates where people
attack the New Testament Scriptures and completely
ignore the Old Testament. We must consider the *entire*
canon of Scripture and obey what it says, regardless
if we like it or not.

2. The Bible proves this notion that all the laws in
Leviticus are limited to the ancient Israelites false.
Homosexuality was sinful for Sodom and Gomorrah,
which were destroyed for their perversion long before
Moses was even born. Homosexuality was also sinful
for the nations who inhabited the land before the
Israelites took possession of it. In Leviticus 18 (the
same chapter God condemned homosexuality), He
explains all the aforementioned sexually deviant acts
in that chapter were also sinful to the other nations
who previously practiced them. These acts were even
sinful to the aliens who lived among the Israelites,
which prove these sexual laws were moral in nature
and thus apply to everyone.

God said, "Do not defile yourselves in any of
these ways, because this is how the nations
that I am going to drive out before you
became defiled. Even the land was defiled;
so I punished it for its sin, and the land vomited out its inhabitants. But you must keep my

decrees and my laws. *The native-born and the aliens living among you must not do any of these detestable things, for all these things were done by the people who lived in the land before you*, and the land became defiled. And if you defile the land, it will vomit you out as it vomited out the nations that were before you. *Everyone who does any of these detestable things*—such persons must be cut off from their people. Keep my requirements and do not follow any of the detestable customs *that were practiced before you came and do not defile yourselves with them.* I am the LORD your God" (Leviticus 18:24-30).

3.  None of God's commandments can be dismissed based on unrelated commandments. The only time we can disregard God's commands is when God himself commands us to do so. For example, there were all sorts of dietary restrictions listed in the book of Leviticus as a part of the Ceremonial Law; however, Jesus ratified these commands in the New Testament when He explained what it was that made a man clean or unclean. In Mark 7:18–19, Jesus says, "Don't you see that nothing that enters a man from the outside can make him 'unclean'? For it doesn't go into his heart but into his stomach, and then out of his body" (In saying this, Jesus declared all foods "clean.") This is reiterated in the book of Acts where Jesus told Peter, "Kill and eat." When Peter refused and said he'd never eaten anything impure or unclean, Jesus replied and said, "Do not call anything impure that God has made clean" (Acts 10:13-15). Therefore, anyone who tries to dredge up any Old Testament Scripture regarding our diet (or any other subject unrelated to sexual

immorality), in an attempt to excuse homosexuality, has failed to understand the entirety of Scripture.

In the event that there is still contention over this issue you can try a different approach. An easy way to dismantle this misunderstanding of Scripture is to simply ask, "Is it sinful for Christians today to have sex with animals?" If you are dealing with an honest person, they will quickly admit bestiality is indeed sinful. Then you can simply ask them, "Where does the Bible condemn bestiality for Christians?" Chances are they won't know how to answer because bestiality is never directly condemned in the New Testament. You can then point out that even though bestiality isn't condemned for Christians in the New Testament, it is repeatedly condemned in Leviticus but the command still holds true for Christians today. This shatters their entire argument by proving there are commands in Leviticus that absolutely do apply to Christians today, which refutes the claim that we must dismiss the entire book of Leviticus.

Concerning the Scripture in the first chapter of Romans, the common accusation is the Apostle Paul wasn't actually talking about homosexuality. A friend of mine who was a religion major at a Christian college first presented this allegation to me. What she was taught concerning this Scripture in Romans is appalling. A group of us debated homosexuality online after Barack Obama suddenly changed his position from supporting "traditional marriage" to promoting homosexuality and "gay marriage." My friend chimed in, letting us all know her credentials as a religion major and then claimed Paul didn't condemn homosexuality; he condemned acts of predation, sexual slaves, prostitution, and other sexual sins. Her entire argument had been copied and pasted from some unnamed source, and essentially alleged that when Paul said "men also abandoned natural relations with women and were inflamed with lust for one another. Men committed indecent acts with other men . . ." that he referred to the abundance of predation at that time between adult males and adolescent males.

In my rebuttal I explained why that interpretation makes no sense at all. The Apostle Paul didn't say, "Men committed indecent acts with *young* men," he said "*other* men," and they were inflamed with lust for "*one another.*" This clearly shows that those engaging in these "homosexual" acts were willful participants. Further, I pointed out that she totally disregarded Paul's condemnation of female homosexuality. Remember, he said, "Even their women exchanged natural relations for unnatural ones. In the same way" that the men did. "*In the same way.*" This is key for two reasons.

First, it clearly shows Paul did not refer to pederasty. Pederasty by definition is the sexual relationship between men and boys. The Greek word that pederasty is derived from literally means "lover of boys." So if this Scripture were about pederasty, it would be self-contradictory because pederasty does not depict sexual relationships between women and girls. In no way does this Scripture imply that females practiced predation and the males practiced predation in the same way. Homosexuality was obviously the topic.

Second, this Scripture proves homosexuality is wrong for both females and males. This is important because some people believe the Bible only condemns male homosexuality but not "lesbianism." This is false. Beyond this, if there is any lingering doubt that homosexuality wasn't prevalent in ancient Rome and Paul condemned pederasty instead, all one must do is examine Roman history, particularly the accounts of the Romans themselves. Early Roman poets, writers, and historians all confirm while pederasty was prevalent in ancient Rome, homosexuality (consenting sexual relationships between two men, and two women) was widely accepted and practiced as well. There are even records of several homosexual weddings taking place describing how one man would play the role of the groom and the other would play the role of the bride and would even wear a wedding veil. These undeniable facts, coupled with Paul's crystal clear condemnation of homosexuality in the book of Romans, totally nullify the false claim he only condemned pederasty.

To my astonishment, my friend replied, not by copying and pasting more content from her unnamed source, but by simply saying, "I respectfully disagree, as I see no valid biblical basis to support that love between men or between women is wrong. Just personal interpretation." Did you catch what happened there? Notice first that after presenting all of my valid fact-based arguments, which clearly proved the Bible does indeed condemn homosexuality, instead of conceding or offering a compelling counterargument, my friend opted to use deflection by claiming *she still didn't see* what the Bible clearly says. Secondly, notice all of the personal pronouns my friend suddenly added. She inadvertently showed her hand by revealing the truth behind her belief: her position wasn't based on what the Bible actually says. Her position was based on *herself*, what *she* saw in the Scripture, and how *she* personally interpreted the Scripture. This is a perfect example of how dangerous irrationality is. It also illustrates exactly how people attempt to modify God's Word and take things way out of context to fit their beliefs, instead of simply reading what God's Word actually says and obeying it. Once again, because we're talking about the Moral Law, the commands on homosexuality apply to *all mankind*. This means it doesn't matter how the Scripture appeared to my friend or how *she* interpreted it; the Scripture still condemns homosexuality. In other words, God's Word doesn't change in order to conform to us; we must change in order to conform to God's Word.

Finally, the challenge commonly brought against the New Testament Scriptures on homosexuality focus on the term "homosexual offender" in 1 Corinthians 6:9 and "homosexuality" in 1 Timothy 1:10. Specifically, the issue is the fact that the Greek word the Apostle Paul used was a word he coined, which is not found elsewhere in Scripture. One common objection is: "There are other more appropriate Greek words the Apostle Paul could have used if he was talking about homosexuality, but he didn't, so it's obvious he wasn't talking about homosexuality." This too is a weak argument that can easily be dismissed once we look at the Greek. The term in question is *arsenokoites,* and to discover the origin of the word and its true definition, one must simply turn to credible references to prove there is nothing cryptic here. According to *Strong's Concordance,* the definition of *arsenokoites* is: "A male engaging in same-gender sexual activity; a sodomite, pederast." According to *Thayer's Greek-English Lexicon of the New Testament*, the definition of *arsenokoites* is: "One who lies with a male as with a female, a sodomite." The definition given by *HELPS Word-studies* is: "A man in bed with another man; a homosexual."

As if that wasn't evidence enough, we can glean even more from the origin of the term. Where did Paul come up with this unique word? We must remember the book of Leviticus was originally written in Hebrew, Paul was fluent in both Hebrew and Greek, Paul was an expert in Old Testament law, and Paul wrote his New Testament letters in Greek. Therefore, the Greek term Paul coined is not random; *arsenokoites* is a deliberate reference to the original Hebrew text. Paul simply translated the Hebrew words in Leviticus describing a man lying with another man into Greek and joined the words together. The result is a word with the exact same meaning that we find in Leviticus. In today's vernacular we simply don't use the phrase, "a man who lies with other men as one lies with women," we say "homosexual" or use the term homosexuality. In other words, "practicing homosexual" is the English equivalent to *arsenokoites*, Paul's Greek translation of the Hebrew text in Leviticus. The three translations not only share the exact same definition, but the recipients of the text knew exactly what was meant as well.

As clearly as we understand the words "homosexual" and homosexuality today, the Gentiles understood Paul's use of the term *arsenokoites*, and the ancient Hebrews understood Moses' description of men who lie with other men as one lies with a woman. Therefore, the challenges brought against Paul's choice of words are baseless, because the meaning of his terminology is consistent across the Old Testament and the New Testament. So with the clarity of the biblical terminology regarding homosexuality no longer in question, these Scriptures can't simply be dismissed as being mistranslated or misinterpreted.

For those determined to blend Christianity and homosexuality together, the only remaining option is to purposefully change what the Bible actually says. This brings us to the creation of the "Gay Bible," formally known as the Queen James Bible. The Queen James Bible is essentially a King James Bible that has twisted each of the Bible verses I've previously referenced regarding homosexuality. What they've done is nothing scholarly. Their objective had nothing to do with the accurate translation of the ancient languages. It was simply a blatant attempt to pretend the Bible approves of homosexuality and to convince others to believe this fabrication. In fact, this maneuver is so blatant the anonymous crafters of the Queen James Bible tell on themselves in their own description of their work. "The Queen James Bible is based on The King James Bible, edited to prevent homophobic misinterpretation . . . We edited those eight verses in a way that makes homophobic interpretations impossible."[25] Notice they did not *translate* these Scriptures from the original languages in which they were written; they *edited* the translation. Specifically, they added words, changed words, and deleted words with total disregard to the original languages so these Scriptures read the way they wish they were actually written.

Their focus was not on accuracy, which is clear in that the editors of this "Bible" remain anonymous. This is because these editors are clearly not scholars in the ancient languages with the credentials to make such edits. They claim their purpose for doing so was to prevent "homophobic misinterpretation," but that is just a smokescreen. Their intent was twofold: to remove the primary source of contention regarding the immorality of homosexuality (the Bible) so Christians can no longer rely on the source of their beliefs, and to appease practicing "homosexuals" and advocates by providing them with a "Bible" that aids them in rationalizing their anti-biblical position. What's most interesting is that even after twisting the aforementioned Scriptures on homosexuality to their liking, none of these edits actually say homosexuality is acceptable or moral behavior. What's more, they failed to edit all the other Scriptures on sexual immorality, purity, marriage, lust, and self-control, all of which oppose homosexuality because homosexuality falls outside the parameters God set for all of those things.

Considering this, we can have every confidence in the actual Bible because credible scholars trained in the ancient languages have translated it accurately. We have also seen any challenge against biblical truth utterly fails, especially attempts as desperate and blatant as those made by the anonymous editors of the Queen James "Bible."

## Conclusion

We have now closely examined the top ten arguments that attempt to prove that homosexuality is not sinful, and we have dismantled them all by proving they are all logically fallacious. At this point it would be wise to pause for a moment and simply consider how God Himself would respond to these arguments. Those people who approve of homosexuality in spite of what the Bible says, and make statements such as, "That's between them and God," also have to answer to God. What will they say when God asks why they supported and approved of those who oppose Him? What will the practicing "homosexuals," who claimed to be Christians and yet ignored the Bible, say to God when they face Him on the Day of Judgment? Do they actually think telling God, "I was born this way," or "The Scriptures about homosexuality were misinterpreted," or "Jesus never spoke against homosexuality," will convince God to allow them to enter heaven? Do they think God will scratch His head and say, "Good point. Come on in to eternal life"? Obviously not. Wisdom says to do everything we can while we can to be righteous and to please God in all our ways. It is simply not worth it to sacrifice eternal bliss with God for a few years of sinful pleasure that will result in eternal destruction.

# 4

# Is Homosexuality Sinful?
# The "Yes" Position

**I**' ve presented a "yes or no question": *is homosexuality sinful?* We began by considering "no" as the first possible answer and examined the most popular arguments "homosexuals" and advocates offer as proof. Since all of these arguments were shown to be irrational and logically fallacious, they were all dismissed. While some might already be convinced that the answer to the question is automatically "yes," in fairness we must consider the arguments for the affirmative with the same scrutiny that we used to examine the arguments for the negative. If in the end we are able to present a logical, rational argument for the affirmative (which the negative failed to do), *then* we will have proven the answer to the question is unequivocally, "Yes. Homosexuality is sinful."

Where then shall we begin? Considering that all the previous arguments we've examined were illogical, let's begin with what a logical argument actually is. A logical argument is a set of premises that, if true, lead to an inescapable conclusion. The premises are like building blocks upon which the conclusion rests. Put simply, a proper logical argument is structured like so: point one is true, point two is true, and point three is true, therefore X conclusion is true. Is it possible to present a valid logical argument that proves that homosexuality is indeed sinful? Yes it is. In fact, it is possible to present several. I've devised two that I will offer for consideration.

## The Moral Argument for the Sinfulness of Homosexuality

The *Moral Argument for the Sinfulness of Homosexuality* is fairly simple. It states:

1. Morality is objective because God authored the Moral Law.
2. The Moral Law embodies God's commandments in the Bible.
3. The Bible expressly condemns homosexuality.
4. Homosexuality is therefore sinful.

In contrast to the previous premises offered in an attempt to prove homosexuality is not sinful, here you can see that we actually have a logical argument that is a progression from contingent premises, which, if all proven true, substantiate the conclusion. Each premise is void of irrationality. The relationship between each premise is logically sound and focuses on the issue at hand, which is *morality,* and the conclusion flows necessarily from the premises that precede it. Now then, if someone was to disagree with the conclusion, they would not only have to dismantle this argument by proving each premise to be false, they would then need to construct a better argument in favor of homosexuality. In all my years discussing and debating homosexuality, this has never happened and I'm confident it never will. Nevertheless, let's not take the premises and conclusion of my logical argument to be true at face value. Let's examine each line one at a time to see *if* they are indeed true, and if so, determine *why* they are true.

## Examining the Logical Argument

**1. Morality is objective because God authored the Moral Law.**
To fully understand this premise, we must be clear on the definitions of the terms within this premise.

*Morality:* the standard of good and right human behavior.
*Objective:* independent of personal feelings, opinions, or interpretations; fact based.
*Subjective:* dependent on personal feelings, opinions, or interpretations; opinion based.
*Moral Law:* The law by which we distinguish between good and evil, and right and wrong human behavior

### Objective Morality
Morality is either objective or subjective. It cannot be neither; it cannot be both. How can we be certain morality is objective and not subjective? This is a rather simple task now that we've clearly defined the terms. Virtually everyone would agree good and evil exist. If good and evil exist, it immediately follows that certain actions are good and certain actions are evil; certain actions are right and certain actions are wrong. Further, because it is impossible for good to be evil and for evil to be good, it is impossible for *good actions* to be evil and for *evil actions* to be good. The two are always

mutually exclusive. To illustrate this point simply we must only examine one example of good and one example of evil. Consider rescuing a drowning child and rape. The former is good and is impossible to be evil no matter how many people say or believe otherwise. The latter is evil and is impossible to be good no matter how many people say or believe otherwise. In the same way, something is not right because we *think* it's right, or we *believe* it's right, or we *want* it to be right. Something is right because it literally *is* right. Thus it is always right to rescue a drowning child and it is always evil to rape someone. Objective morality is as simple as saying 1 + 1 = 2 is true. Even if everyone in the world decided 1 + 1 = 3, 1 + 1 = 2 would still be true.

Objective morality is universal—it applies to all mankind, it transcends mankind, it is absolute, flawless, and unchanging. Put plainly, when it comes to objectivity, opinions are irrelevant. The truth of morality endures regardless of how we feel or what we think about it. In fact, there are two ways to easily summarize objective morality. The first is a simple statement: *right is right even if everyone believes it is wrong, and wrong is wrong even if everyone believes it is right.* The second is to envision it.

**FIGURE 2**
Objective Morality

The image you see here is a visual representation of objective morality. Half of the image is perfectly black, and the other is perfectly white with a sharp line of contrast going down the center. This is a simple but accurate reflection of objective morality. There is good and evil, right and wrong, godliness and ungodliness; one is completely contrary to the other, and the distinction is absolute even if we are confused, deceived, blind, or never looked at this image.

### Subjective Morality

Subjective morality is a contradictory concept that is primarily held by atheists. Atheists are well aware if God exists, objective morality exists, and since they deny God's existence, they must also deny the existence of objective morality. The classical Moral Argument is powerful evidence for God's existence. It says simply:

1. If God does not exist, objective moral values and duties do not exist.
2. Objective moral values and duties exist.
3. Therefore God exists.

Atheists generally agree with the first premise, and since they already deny the conclusion, which is that God exists, they must therefore deny the second premise, which is that objective morality exists. Otherwise, their worldview would be even less plausible considering the strong lack of evidence to support it. In any case, if objective morality does not exist, only two alternatives remain for the atheists to maintain their position: subjective morality, or the denial of morality altogether. To deny morality altogether is a silly notion because sooner or later the anti-moralist always tells on himself by making a moral affirmation.

We find an example of this in the militant atheist Richard Dawkins. On one hand, Dawkins, in one of his most famous quotes, claims, "The universe we observe has precisely the properties we should expect if there is, at bottom, no design, no purpose, no evil and no good, nothing but blind pitiless indifference."[26] Then on the other hand he claims, "Faith is one of the world's great evils, comparable to the smallpox virus but harder to eradicate."[27] Of course, the irony is Dawkins has faith this statement is true, which is a contradiction in itself, but more importantly this statement identifies faith as "evil," which totally contradicts his claim that there is no evil. Can you see the foolishness here? So as we've said, good and evil exist, which easily repudiates the idea that morality doesn't exist.

Subjective moralists recognize good and evil do in fact exist; however, they fail to recognize the glaring flaws in their position. In contrast to objective morality, subjective morality is dependent on opinions, feelings, and interpretations; it is not universal (it does not apply to all mankind – it is limited to the subject), it does not transcend mankind, it is not absolute, it is not flawless, and it is not unchanging. This concept of morality obviously contradicts the very nature of morality. In fact, subjective morality violates one of the fundamental laws of classical logic known as the *law of noncontradiction*. This law states that it is impossible for contradictory statements to hold true at the same time and in the same context. In other words, it's impossible for rape to be good and evil simultaneously, and yet subjective moralists believe otherwise.

I actually had a debate with an atheist who refused to acknowledge morality is objective because he knew that doing so would disprove his atheistic worldview. His responses to my questions about rape were astonishing. He said his personal opinion was that rape was bad but that didn't mean it was universally wrong. This is an absolutely absurd statement especially coming from someone who was never raped – it's easy to say rape is morally right in some situations when you've never been in that horrible situation. I then personalized my inquiry by asking if it would be wrong if *he* were the rape victim. His responded, "Rape is not objectively wrong. It is subjectively good or bad according to the taste of the individual." Can you believe that? In other words, rape is morally wrong for the victim but morally right for the rapist! This is just one illustration of the utter foolishness of subjective morality.

Of the litany of flaws inherent in the concept of subjective morality, two are paramount. First is the misperception that having and voicing one's opinion about morality literally affects morality. This idea defies both logic and common sense. If this were true, when I say that rape is wrong, then rape becomes morally wrong because that's my opinion. However, when someone else says that rape is right, then rape becomes morally right because that's their opinion. So what is moral and immoral is in constant flux depending on who is voicing their opinion. This is clearly a ridiculous notion. Subjective morality is not true morality; it is merely one's *opinion about* morality. Subjective morality is limited to the mind, which explains why it cannot possibly apply to anyone beyond the subject. Further, one must simply use common sense to see how this view fails. Words have meanings, and the definition of good includes words such as excellent, virtuous, beneficent, and pious. In contrast, the definition of evil includes words such as wicked, harmful, vicious, and cruel. Thus, common sense dictates that when someone says rape is good, it is clear that they are deceived or lying because rape does not fit the definition of good in any way. It does, however, perfectly fit the definition of evil. This clearly shows that a person's opinion simply has no affect whatsoever on morality because morality exists outside the mind – which proves that it is objective. Therefore, if an individual's opinion cannot possibly affect morality, then a majority's opinion cannot possibly affect morality. In fact, even a universal opinion fails to affect morality because morality transcends human opinion.

The second fundamental flaw in subjective morality is that it is grounded in nothing. Atheists can offer no intelligible source upon which their concept of morality is grounded. Without a valid reference point, how can one person's moral opinion supersede another person's moral opinion? Surely the man who affirms it is morally right to kill innocent Americans and the man who affirms it is morally wrong to kill innocent Americans aren't both correct. It's either one or the other. Yet without a moral basis, subjective morality fails to determine which moral affirmation is valid. Subjective morality essentially means, "anything goes." Anything at anytime can be considered moral or immoral by anyone, and nobody else can overrule them. So what does subjective morality look like?

**FIGURE 3**
Subjective Morality

The image you see here is a visual representation of subjective morality. This time, instead of a sharp contrast between black and white, there's a gradient between black on the far left and white on the far right with the majority of the image filled with tones of gray. In this case, what you see is literally a gray area between the two extremes. It's impossible to distinguish between what is good and what is evil, what is right and what is wrong, because it's all a blend of the two extremes. Everything is a matter of perception or taste based on the individual's feelings, opinions, and interpretations.

To make this distinction clear, let's consider another real-life example: under the rules of subjective morality a man can assert that cheating on his wife is not immoral because he is no longer attracted to her, and so he has numerous adulterous relationships. His wife can then assert that because her husband cheated on her, there is nothing immoral with retaliating by cheating on him. The husband, however, can then assert that his wife is immoral for cheating. Do you see how nonsensical this concept of morality is? Subjective morality makes it impossible to determine who is actually right and who is wrong when there is a moral conflict. On the contrary, objective morality says adultery is wrong at any time, under any circumstance, for *everyone*. The difference is quite clear, and it is also clear why some people would prefer subjective morality to objective morality.

When we step back and are completely honest with ourselves, we will discover there are two primary reasons for accepting subjective morality over objective morality: to support the belief that God doesn't exist, and to attempt to free oneself of moral accountability. As such, those who try to convince themselves that morality is subjective don't do so on account of any factual evidence, but because they *want* morality to be subjective. If morality is objective that means God exists and there are rules fixed in place that we must follow in order to be moral. This poses an immediate problem for those who wish to be free of all moral accountability because this makes it difficult to behave however they please without the burden of feeling guilty. Subjective moralists essentially say, "I don't like the moral standards God has set (or I don't like that idea that God exists), so I'll set my own moral standards, which I reserve the right to change whenever I like depending on how I feel at the time." They try to convince themselves that they are moral authorities—they have the power to set the rules of good and right human behavior and exempt themselves from answering to anyone for their actions. This is precisely how people rationalize gratifying their sinful desires: "It might be wrong for you, but it's not wrong for me." This is as foolish as saying, "That color might be black to you, but it is white to me." Of course, black is never white, and white is never black so this obviously does absolutely nothing to disprove objective morality. Merely ignoring objective morality doesn't make it disappear, nor does reshaping it in one's mind alter it in any way. Yet this is precisely what atheists and other subjective moralists believe happens.

Every time an atheist makes a moral affirmation declaring something is wrong, we must only ask them, "Why? How do you know that it's wrong? On what basis are you making that claim?" We will receive no acceptable answer because once again, in atheism there is *no valid basis for morality.* Atheists believe we're merely products of evolution; they believe humans are essentially animals, but animals are not free moral agents. Morality doesn't exist in the animal kingdom; it's merely survival of the fittest. Humans, however, are free moral agents. How can this be without a moral authority that serves as a starting point, the source and standard upon which morality rests? It cannot. Subjective morality by its definition is irrational—unclear thinking based on *opinions* and *feelings,* not on facts and reason—it lacks the foundation or source necessary to validate it or even make it plausible, and it violates the law of noncontradiction. Consequently, any moral framework built outside of objective morality is flawed from its core and riddled with folly and deception. We can therefore confidently assert that anyone who claims morality is subjective is either confused or lying. Good and evil existed before mankind existed. How then can anyone who was born *after* good and evil presume to dictate what is good and what is evil? After that person dies, what happens to those customized moral affirmations? Surely they don't apply to all mankind. Surely they don't endure indefinitely. The fact is no one can affect morality. Because morality precedes mankind and it is grounded in God – the object and Author of the Moral Law, it stands alone and transcends mankind – the subject. In other words, morality flows from a singular perfect source, which is God, not from billions of imperfect humans. Because humans are not perfect or all-knowing, we are capable and often guilty of being ignorant, confused, and deceived. Thus anyone who attempts to dictate the parameters of morality from this flawed position simply cannot be trusted as an authoritative moral lawgiver. We all can relate to this. Every one of us, at some point in our lives, were absolutely convinced a certain action we took was righteous, but in time we came to the realization that we were mistaken and that action was absolutely unrighteous. In fact, in many cases these moral deceptions occur more often than not. This fallible condition discounts every human from establishing what is good and evil, and right and wrong for mankind. Only a perfect being (one who is incapable of making errors), an all-knowing being (one who is incapable of being ignorant, confused, or deceived), and a perfectly moral being (one who is incapable of lying or doing evil) can establish the Moral Law, because that is the only way the Law would be perfect and binding for all mankind. This proves the objectivity of morality.

### *Moral Law*

It is one thing to understand *that* morality is objective; it is another to understand *why* morality is objective. The reason objective morality is universal, transcendent, absolute, flawless, and unchanging is because the Author of the Moral Law is universal, transcendent, absolute, flawless, and unchanging. Therefore, the Moral Law flows naturally from God and is binding because He is the only perfect moral agent.

What else do we know about God? God is good by definition. He is love, He is righteous, He is perfect, He is truth, He is just, He is all-powerful, and He is all-knowing. God isn't good in the sense that He behaves well; He literally *is* good. In fact, He is goodness in its highest form. So naturally anything outside of God's goodness is evil. God is the highest form of righteousness. So naturally anything outside of God's righteousness is unrighteous. God is the highest form of love. So naturally anything outside of God's love is not love. Because God is all-knowing and just, His commands are always perfect and good. Therefore, whatever God says is good, *is good*, and whatever God says is evil, *is evil*. This is undeniable because God is incapable of lying, He knows all things, and He cannot make mistakes. This is why Proverbs 3:5 commands us: "Trust in the Lord with all your heart and lean not on your own understanding." Why? We cannot trust in our own understanding because we are not all-knowing. God is. So regardless if we understand God's Moral Law or not, it doesn't matter; we're obligated to trust in Him because He is righteous and trustworthy. This is why we can have every confidence that God's Moral Law is good and perfect, and because God's Moral Law is good and perfect, morality is necessarily objective.

## 2. The Moral Law embodies God's commandments in the Bible.

God communicates to us in many ways, but the one that is most easily recognizable is the Bible. The Bible is God's inerrant Word. It not only boasts this claim for itself, it proves this claim by its accuracy, authority, and authenticity. Moreover, God's biblical commands are perfectly consistent with what we know of morality and our moral experience. There is not one biblical command that defies morality because it is based on morality. Consider a few commandments of the Moral Law in the Old Testament: love God, don't be an idolater, honor your parents, don't murder, don't be sexually immoral, don't commit adultery, don't steal, don't lie, and don't be envious. Or a few listed in the New Testament: don't be sexually immoral, don't be impure, don't be hateful, jealous, or selfish, don't be a drunkard. Every single commandment of the Moral Law from the Old Testament through the New Testament is good in itself because it came from God, but it also produces goodness in us by obeying it. The gamut of moral behavior is addressed in the Bible, and God's commands make it perfectly clear what is good and right behavior, and what is evil and wrong behavior.

### 3. The Bible expressly condemns homosexuality.
This has already been proven by examining the Old Testament and New Testament Scriptures that specifically address homosexuality, and beyond this there are twenty-seven Scriptures on sexual immorality in addition to all the other Scriptures on marriage, love, lust, purity, evil thoughts, and self-control—all of which apply to homosexuality. Although many people, including those who falsely claim to be Christians, try to make it seem like the Bible is not crystal clear on homosexuality, the truth is the Bible couldn't be any clearer on homosexuality without being graphic. The Bible spells it out repeatedly in various ways, and not once does it approve of homosexuality in any way.

### 4. Homosexuality is therefore sin.
This brings us to the inescapable conclusion that yes, homosexuality is indeed sinful. Keep in mind that disliking or disagreeing with this conclusion is irrelevant. Opinions or feelings don't disprove logically sound arguments, nor do they alter God's commands. If we have a problem with God or His word, the fault is never with God but always with us. Whatever God says is true and binding as the Psalmist says of God: "All your words are true; all your righteous laws are

eternal" (Psalm 119:160). We can therefore say with confidence that homosexuality is a violation of God's Moral Law, because He said it was.

## Challenging the Moral Argument

Unfortunately, scores of professing Christians ignore the logic and rationality of this powerful argument. They reject this truth, declaring, "I still don't *believe* homosexuality is a sin," or "I still don't *agree* homosexuality is a sin," or "I still don't *understand* how homosexuality is a sin." All those responses are based on *them,* and *their opinions,* not on *God* and His *perfect and eternal Moral Law.* Remember, when it comes to objectivity opinions are irrelevant. With this in mind, it becomes quite clear these declarations are all subjective and blatant violations of God's command in Proverbs 3:5 to trust in Him with all our hearts and lean *not* on our own understanding. If a professing Christian reaches this point and still chooses to reject the truth that homosexuality is sinful, the good news is that they don't have to be a Christian. No one is forcing them to claim Christianity and follow God's commands. That is the beauty of free will. But they can't try to get the benefits of Christianity while agreeing with and practicing sin because that doesn't work. Christianity opposes sinfulness, it does not ignore or embrace sinfulness. Those that disagree have every right to ignore and reject God, but that doesn't mean there are no consequences for doing so. To reject God's Word is to reject God, which is to reject the solution to all their problems, along with the blessings, protection, grace, and favor that come through obedience to God. On top of all that, in rejecting God they are also rejecting His free gift of salvation. Thus, it would be wise to stop agreeing with that which is sinful, stop promoting it, clinging to it, and indulging in it, and cling to life and the Giver of eternal life instead.

It addition to professing Christians who will try to rebut this argument, you will most likely encounter an unbeliever who will respond to this argument by saying, "Well, I'm not a Christian. God does not exist," and they will often proceed to attack God, the Bible, or you. Or perhaps all three—I've had that happen before. At this point you can opt to defend God, the Bible, and yourself, or you can move directly to the second logical argument. If you choose the former, I recommend presenting the classical arguments for God's existence. I've already shared the classical Moral Argument for God's existence, but there are several more. The Kalam Cosmological Argument, the Fine Tuning Argument, and the Argument from the Historicity of Jesus Christ are all powerful logical arguments that point to God's existence. These arguments taken collectively are too formidable for any honest, logical thinker to deny. Atheists have no such logical arguments. They simply rely on trying to tear these arguments down (which fails) but never construct logical arguments in place of these that point powerfully toward God's nonexistence. It will take some time and research, but I highly recommend all Christians become familiar with these arguments and be fully capable of presenting powerful arguments in favor of God's existence to anyone at any time. This is not just a good idea, this is a command as we find in 1 Peter 3:15: "Always be prepared to give an answer to everyone who asks you to give the reason for the hope that you have, but do this with gentleness and respect." I've given you a starting point for defending the validity and authenticity of the Bible. I also recommend that you do some credible research and be prepared to defend any attacks against the Bible with factual evidence. I'm certain you are well prepared to defend yourself, because if you've been a Christian for any considerable amount of time, you have already done so repeatedly and will continue to do so.

# The Natural Argument for the Immorality of Homosexuality

Even if someone refuses to accept the concept of God and/ or Christianity, that doesn't mean that homosexuality isn't immoral, nor are you out of options in proving your position. Remember there are *two* logical arguments that I've devised, and at this point we've only considered one. In the event that someone adamantly rejects the *Moral Argument for the Sinfulness of Homosexuality* despite failing to prove it false, you can run the *Natural Argument for the Immorality of Homosexuality.* "Sinful" and "immoral" are synonyms so this argument works well for those who deny God's existence and refuse to acknowledge the reality of sin. The wonderful thing about the natural argument is that it is not only logical, rational, and simple, but most people already agree with the first premise. Even if they disagree with the second, they can easily be convinced this premise is also true after reviewing the overwhelming amount of evidence that proves it. Thus, the conclusion that logically follows is inescapable. So let's look at *The Natural Argument for the Immorality of Homosexuality:*

1. It is immoral to harm yourself, to harm others, or to subject yourself or others to harm.
2. Because homosexuality is unnatural it is harmful to all parties involved.
3. Therefore homosexuality is immoral.

As I've said, you can almost guarantee that after asking the simple question, "Would you agree that it's immoral to harm yourself, to harm others, or to subject yourself or others to harm?" anyone with common sense will answer "yes." Chances are the second premise will immediately be challenged. At this point, it would be helpful to have a few facts prepared in order to prove homosexuality is indeed harmful to all parties involved. The fact concerning the harmfulness of homosexuality remains: *the rates for sexually transmitted diseases, promiscuity, substance abuse (drug and alcohol), violence, depression, suicide, cancer, abuse (mental, psychological, sexual), infidelity, physical damage, mental health distress, and mortality are all drastically higher in the "homosexual" community as compared to the "heterosexual" community.* Remember, this is not speculation or an opinion. This is a proven fact. I'll provide a few statistics as proof, but I encourage you to consult some quality resources to see for yourself the factual evidence that shows how harmful and dangerous the "homosexual" lifestyle is.

- Sexually Transmitted Diseases (STDs) have been increasing among gay and bisexual men, with recent increases in syphilis being documented across the country. In 2012, men who have sex with men (MSM) accounted for seventy-five percent of primary and secondary syphilis cases in the United States. MSM often are diagnosed with other STDs, including chlamydia and gonorrhea infections.[28]
- Seventy-five percent of "homosexual" men carry one or more sexually transmitted diseases, *wholly apart* from AIDS.[29]
- Women who have sexual relations with women (WSW) are at significantly higher risk for certain sexually transmitted diseases: "We demonstrated a higher prevalence of bv (bacterial vaginosis), hepatitis C,

and HIV risk behaviors in WSW as compared with controls."[30]

- In a survey of 1,099 lesbians, the *Journal of Social Service Research* found "slightly more than half of the [lesbians] reported that they had been abused by a female lover/partner. The most frequently indicated forms of abuse were verbal/emotional/psychological abuse and combined physical-psychological abuse."[31]
- The incidence of domestic violence among gay men is nearly double that in the heterosexual population.[32]

Let's examine a few of these negative effects of homosexuality a little closer. There are over twenty types of STDs, and millions and millions of Americans are infected every single year. We mustn't forget while there are *treatments* for some of the most common and most lethal STDs such as HIV/AIDS, HPV, and genital herpes, there are no *cures* for these diseases. They are highly contagious and therefore highly dangerous in the general population. The fact that these diseases are far more prevalent in the "homosexual" community is alarming and simply can't be ignored.

As mentioned earlier, many people are unaware of the significance promiscuity has in the "homosexual" community. Monogamy and fidelity are rarities in both "gay" and "lesbian" relationships. As we've seen, because of the compulsive and addictive nature of homosexuality, "homosexuals" are known to have had hundreds of sexual partners, while a significant number have even had a thousand or more sexual partners. This doesn't always change when "homosexuals" enter committed relationships. The fact is "homosexuals" rarely find satisfaction in one partner, so "gay" couples commonly agree to an open relationship instead of a sexually exclusive relationship. This is obviously wrought with problems, which lead to many of the other negative effects I've listed.

Substance abuse often accentuates sexual experiences, but it also dulls the mind, which leads to foolish decisions. This results in wilder and riskier sexual encounters, which in turn lead to STD infections and a range of other negative results such as violence, abuse, and mental health distress. I've read "homosexuals" were more susceptible to cancer compared to "heterosexuals." This seemed odd to me because I did not understand the correlation between homosexuality and cancer. Further research proved the biblical statement of two "becoming one flesh" is not merely a reference to a husband and wife consummating marriage by having sex, but it is a literal depiction of what happens on a cellular level during "heterosexual" intercourse. The female immune system is complex. When a foreign substance enters a woman's body, her immune system immediately identifies that substance as foreign and rejects it. This would prove to be problematic for conceiving children if it weren't for the brilliant way God designed males and females. When a male's seminal fluid enters a woman's body, a component hardcoded inside the sperm sends signals to the woman's body. These signals allow the sperm to be accepted instead of identified as a foreign body and rejected by the woman's immune system. When this happens the woman literally accepts the seminal fluid as part of her own body. In this way the two become one flesh.[33] Now, what happens when this process is violated and males have sexual relations with other males? When semen is deposited into another male, the signals that are hardcoded to communicate with a female's body cannot be interpreted by another male's body. In addition, sperm is designed to penetrate a female's egg, which results in conception. Sperm deposited into another male's body don't understand that they are in the wrong body and still behave the way they are created to. Sperm have the ability to penetrate other cells and overtake the nucleus of those cells. So when sperm enters a male instead of a female, cells within the male's body are often penetrated and overtaken. When this happens cancerous growths are formed within the male. This is the consequence of an obvious biological violation. Any behavior that causes cancer in other people is undeniably immoral.

Now, men are not the only ones in danger here. There are studies that show a possible link between "lesbianism" and cancer in women too. The most common types of cancer among women are breast, colon, endometrial (uterine), cervical, lung, and skin cancer. Studies have found that "lesbians" and "bisexual" women have higher rates of breast cancer than "heterosexual" women.[34]

In addition to all the infections, diseases, and cancer, there are the multiple ways in which "homosexual" males suffer physical damage, some of which is permanent. Male and female bodies are obviously complementary. Each was designed specifically for the other, together they serve a specific function, and neither suffers physical damage in the process. The rectum is simply not complementary to a male's genitalia. One was not designed specifically for the other. Further, although what follows is graphic, it is important to understand that "homosexual" activity is not limited to what most believe. "Homosexual" males seek gratification in all sorts of lewd and harmful ways using all sorts of foreign objects including live animals. There is even something called "fisting," a pretty self-explanatory sexually activity, which is common in the "homosexual" community. I'm sure you can imagine how much physical damage these illicit behaviors cause. The rectum was specifically designed for one purpose, and that is to rid the body of waste. When it is used for "homosexual" purposes, it causes severe problems, including rectal prolapse, ruptures, multiple parasitic diseases, prostate damage, diarrhea, and chronic fecal incontinence. As a consequence of these harmful effects, "homosexual" males are often forced to wear adult diapers because they are no longer capable of controlling their bowels. I would hope nobody would deny these are conditions no one wants to experience much less endure for the rest of their lives. I would also hope everyone would agree that it is immoral to cause other people to suffer these devastating conditions.

Once again, while many think the negative results of homosexuality are exclusive to males, this isn't true. "Homosexual" females are at higher risk of suffering many of these same effects as compared to "heterosexual" females. The sexual practices "lesbians" engage in, including sex toys and other penetrative means, are capable of causing physical damage and spreading infections and diseases as well. This behavior also accounts for the high rate of STDs in the "homosexual" community. The violence, abuse, and other negative affects previously mentioned also apply to "lesbians." The evidence proving that homosexuality is harmful because it is unnatural is abundantly clear, and we've not yet addressed the profound negative impact homosexuality has on children, families, communities, and societies, which further points to the immoral nature of homosexuality. The inescapable conclusion, even from a strictly natural standpoint, is clear: homosexuality is immoral because it is an unnatural, unhealthy, harmful, and dangerous lifestyle.

## Challenging the Natural Argument

How could anyone deny such an abundance of well-documented facts? With so much unbiased evidence validating the Natural Argument, isn't this clearly an open-and-shut case? Not in some people's minds. There are die-hard supporters of homosexuality who absolutely refuse to accept the truth, even if that requires them to make the nonsensical claim that facts lie. I've actually had skeptics of this caliber send me information from the CDC that supposedly refutes the

Natural Argument. Ironically, these skeptics only skimmed the content they sent because in each case the CDC's findings actually *confirmed* the dangers of homosexuality! The CDC, while not immune to political correctness, finally admitted "gay" and "bisexual" men are in the highest risk group for contracting STDs, a fact that defenders of homosexuality have denied for many years. So these skeptics, in their desperate attempt to disprove the Natural Argument, inadvertently proved it to be accurate. Of course when I reiterated the truth citing their own sources, they had nothing to say in response. Experiences such as these have taught me a valuable lesson: after examining the facts, the truth about homosexuality is obvious even to those who refuse to admit it.

# How to Respond to Skeptics

Presenting logical arguments that prove homosexuality is sinful/immoral will undoubtedly incite rebuttals from obstinate skeptics. How should you respond? First, you must recognize the fallacious nature of their rebuttals. Then you must respond in a respectful way that dismisses their error and reiterates the truth. While this may seem daunting at first, I assure you it's not. You will be more than capable of responding appropriately by knowing what to expect and how to accurately interpret rebuttals. To assist you in this endeavor I've comprised a list of popular rebuttals from skeptics I've had exchanges with over the years. Consider what follows a training exercise and a blueprint to follow going forward. Here's a tip: Misdirection is one of the primary tools skeptics use to challenge opponents of homosexuality. Avoid being distracted by remaining absolutely focused on the topic here, which is the sinfulness/immorality of homosexuality. This will expose the manipulative and deceptive nature of these challenges and teach you how to remain steadfast, rational, and logical in your responses.

**1. "I think good Christians should continue to love and not judge, especially something that they don't understand."** *Logical Fallacy Committed: Red Herring*—introducing an irrelevant topic to shift attention away from the argument.

**Note:** Comments of this sort are a veiled condemnation. There are two implications here. The first is that you are a subpar Christian because you openly oppose homosexuality. In other words, they're saying, "If you were really a good Christian you'd be like me and remain silent on homosexuality." The second implication is that you are ignorant and therefore wrong. What the skeptic is actually saying here is, "I understand homosexuality but you don't, because if you did you wouldn't oppose it." Not only is this mindset flawed, it is meant to distract you from the topic at hand. Don't fall for this trap.

**Appropriate Response:** It's interesting that you condemn judging and yet your entire statement was judgmental. Nevertheless, let's stick to the facts. First, love is not ignoring or enabling our neighbors' sinfulness; love is helping our neighbors abstain from sinfulness. Jesus was dedicated to saving people from sin, and healing both the sick and diseased. Homosexuality is sinful and the cause of many sicknesses and diseases. So naturally Jesus would oppose this behavior if he were here physically. In lieu of this, Christians follow Christ's example by loving "homosexuals" enough to try to save them from this dangerous and sinful lifestyle. Second, Christ never remained silent in the face of sin; He opposed it in all of its forms wherever he went. Christians do likewise. Third, Christ commissioned us to "Go into all the world and preach the good news to all creation." I intend to continue obeying Jesus by helping as many "homosexuals" as I can, and I invite you to join me by doing the same.

**2. "I know you don't keep all the Scriptures so you should focus on your own sins."**
*Logical Fallacy Committed: Red Herring*—introducing an irrelevant topic to shift attention away from the argument.

**Note:** This is actually an indirect concession that homosexuality is sinful, which is a good thing, but it is designed to distract you from the issue. The implication is that everyone leads a sinful lifestyle, which means it's wrong for anyone to oppose homosexuality because only a sinless person would have the right to do such a thing. This implication is false.

**Appropriate Response:** We agree that homosexuality is sinful and that sins should be overcome. However, not everyone lives a sinful lifestyle as you suggest. There is a big difference between an imperfect Christian whose lifestyle is dedicated to avoiding sin, and a sinner whose lifestyle is dedicated to embracing and practicing sin. Christians aren't only concerned for our own salvation; we are also concerned for the salvation of everyone enslaved by sin. As former sinners, Christians are sensitive to the fact that the lost desperately need help. In fact, Jesus commanded us to identify sin and help one another overcome it. So obeying Christ and helping people overcome homosexuality is not only a good thing, it is the right thing to do.

**3. "For [expletive] sake! You're not even worth it."**
*Logical Fallacy Committed: Ad Hominem*—attacking the person instead of addressing the argument.

**Note:** Comments such as this are meant to make you angry and abandon the conversation. However, Proverbs 15:1 says,

"A gentle answer turns away wrath," so even if it takes all the restraint you can muster, avoid responding with anger. You have a choice here: you can attempt to shift the conversation back to an amicable place in order to continue, or you can politely excuse yourself if you're dealing with a belligerent skeptic. You are not obligated to endure hostility, especially if you remained respectful throughout the discourse.

**Appropriate Response 1:** I've shown you nothing but respect and ask that you return the favor. This topic is worth discussing and I would love to continue if you're willing to calm down.

**Appropriate Response 2:** I will continue praying for you. Take care.

## 4. "Keep that venomous closed-minded thinking to yourself."

*Logical Fallacy Committed: Strawman Fallacy*—misrepresenting or fabricating an opponent's argument to make it easier to attack.

**Note:** This is a tactic to silence Christians by maligning the truth in an effort to dismiss the truth. Of course, painting the truth in an ugly light does not make it untrue. In this case, the goal is for you to immediately retract your statement or end the conversation to avoid being labeled a bully, "homophobic," bigoted, etc. You must recognize this deception, stay on topic, and continue to share the truth.

**Appropriate Response:** Surely you aren't suggesting that the truth is venomous? The truth is consistent and impartial. Open-minded people accept the truth whether they like it or not. Closed-minded people reject any truth they dislike. I understand why you don't like the fact that homosexuality is sinful, but that doesn't make it untrue.

**5. "If I'm going to hell because of who I love, I don't want to serve that God."**
***Logical Fallacy Committed:*** *Strawman Fallacy*—misrepresenting or fabricating an opponent's argument to make it easier to attack.

**Note:** There are two things going on here. First, the argument has been purposefully distorted in order to manipulate you. Notice the sinfulness of homosexuality (which is the topic here) was eliminated from the equation and replaced with "love." Fabricating this dire scenario is designed to make you pause and think, *hell certainly seems like a harsh punishment for merely loving someone,* and then start doubting the truth. Don't be deceived by this false notion. Anyone who goes to hell chooses to go to hell by choosing to love *sin* instead of loving *God*. One can either love God and reject sin or love sin and reject God. The two are mutually exclusive and the consequences of each choice are abundantly clear in Scripture. Secondly, this statement, which was actually made by a professing Christian, implies that there are multiple Gods. Apparently this includes one that embraces homosexuality. Obviously this notion is false. There is only one God, His word is eternal, and His word condemns homosexuality as a sinful practice that inevitably leads to eternal destruction.

**Appropriate Response:** True love doesn't justify sin, nor does it lead to sin. If the result of your "love" is sin, then it's not love; it's lust. There is only one God. Rejecting Him and indulging in sin is what sends people to hell. Since homosexuality is sinful, by choosing to love it you reject God. Unless you change and wholeheartedly repent, hell is where the *Bible* says you will go. That is why this conversation is so important. God doesn't want you to go to hell. I don't want you to go to hell, and deep down you don't want to go to hell either. But whether you go to hell or not is entirely up to you.

God sacrificed His only Son to save you from sin and offer you salvation. Why would you choose to ignore that sacrifice to embrace sin and reject God's salvation?

**6. "I know what Scriptures lead me."**
***Logical Fallacy Committed:*** *Confirmation Bias*—relying on evidence that confirms one's preconceived belief while ignoring and/or rejecting all evidence contrary to that belief.

**Note:** This is a statement commonly made by professing Christians who attempt to mix their favorite sin with Christianity and pretend God condones it. They've convinced themselves that they only have to follow the Scriptures they like, but have the right to reject the Scriptures they dislike. This level of deception is dangerous and does not excuse sin of any kind.

**Appropriate Response:** Christians cannot pick and choose which Scriptures they will follow and which ones they won't. That's hypocrisy and there is no hypocrisy in Christianity. Those who serve Christ as Lord obey *all* of God's word, which includes the Scriptures that make them uncomfortable. This means that if you're a Christian, you can't ignore all the Scriptures about homosexuality, sexual immorality, love, lust, purity, and marriage because they don't "lead" you. Either Christ is your Lord and you fully obey his word, or He isn't and you don't.

**7. "As a Christian you know that God doesn't make mistakes. I'm perfect being gay."**
***Logical Fallacy Committed:*** *False Cause*— presuming a relationship between two things means one caused the other.

**Note:** This statement begins with the truth, ends with a lie, and presupposes the latter is the result of the former. The implication here is that God makes people "gay." If that is true, and God doesn't make mistakes, then "gay" people are perfect being "gay." The validity of this argument, however, hinges on whether or not God does indeed make people "gay." He doesn't. The truth is we are all born into sin. Sin manifests itself in many ways and homosexuality is one of those manifestations. Since sin doesn't come from God this entire argument fails. It's also important to point out that no one is perfect aside from God.

**Appropriate Response:** We agree that God does not make mistakes. What you're implying though, is that God makes people "gay." This is not only false, it's impossible because God cannot contradict Himself. It would be a contradiction to establish that homosexuality is sinful, command mankind to abstain from it, and then make people "gay." Further, everyone is imperfect so it's impossible for you to be "perfect being 'gay.'" The good news is we can strive for perfection. The way we do that is by following God's command to abstain from all sins, which includes homosexuality, and by mirroring the life of Jesus Christ—the only perfect person who ever lived.

**8. "That is not true and there are a large number of people who would disagree with you."**
*Logical Fallacy Committed: Appeal to Popularity*—claiming a statement is true or false based solely on a majority consensus.

**Note:** This is a desperate measure. First, it is conjecture—anyone can make this claim about anything; that doesn't make it factual. Second, the majority doesn't determine what is true and what is false. The issue here is not how many people believe homosexuality is not sinful; the issue is whether or not homosexuality is sinful. We have already proven that it is. The truth is in the evidence and disagreeing doesn't change the facts.

**Appropriate Response:** Truth is not determined by popular opinion. Truth persists despite popular opinion. For example, the world didn't become flat because everyone once agreed it was. The factual evidence I've presented is clear and it proves homosexuality is sinful/immoral. If you have any evidence to the contrary, I'll be happy to examine it, but merely saying "that's not true" and appealing to popularity doesn't change the facts.

**9. "Homosexuality is natural. It's found in many animal species so it's natural in humans too."**
*Logical Fallacies Committed: Equivocation*—using the same word with two different meanings to misrepresent the truth; doublespeak. *Appeal to Nature* — the assertion that because something is "natural" it is justified or good.

**Note:** It's critical to understand how this popular argument commits the equivocation fallacy. The word *natural* has several meanings. The two relevant definitions here are: *existing in nature* and *in accordance with nature*. The first pertains to state of being; the second pertains to conformity to design and order. These two definitions are obviously dissimilar and therefore cannot be used interchangeably; yet that is precisely what this argument attempts to do. When interpreted accurately this argument reads: Homosexuality [exists in nature]. It's found in many animal species so it's [in accordance with nature] in humans too. This is clearly the implication because no one denies that homosexuality exists in humans, and the skeptic's objective here is to justify human homosexuality. This implication, however, is plainly false. Although homosexuality exists, it is *not* in accordance with nature. This is why it is unnatural. While homosexuality has allegedly been observed in some animal species, it is an extreme rarity for obvious reasons: life can only be produced through natural sexual behavior, which means homosexuality is detrimental to the survival of the species. Additionally, it's easy to disprove this attempt to justify homosexuality by citing behavior observed in animals. All we must do is consider the plethora of other sexual behaviors that exist in the animal kingdom but are clearly unnatural human behavior. For example, forceful copulation is prevalent in the animal kingdom. There is nothing immoral about this behavior because morality doesn't exist in the animal kingdom. However, rape (the human equivalent) is clearly immoral and unnatural human behavior. So the *existence* of forceful copulation in animals doesn't mean rape is *in accordance with nature* in humans. See the distinction? No one with common sense would ever tell a rape victim that rape is justified human behavior because it's natural in the animal kingdom. One has absolutely nothing to do with the other. Now, if we were to abandon common sense and logic to justify homosexuality through the *Equivocation* fallacy, we would also have to justify the human equivalent to all sorts of bizarre mating practices that have been observed in animals. This would include violent attacks before, during, and after sex; murder; cannibalism; incest; and inbreeding. Obviously it would be absurd to try to justify these behaviors in humans simply because they have been observed in animals. Homosexuality is no exception so it simply cannot be justified in this deceptive fashion. As if that wasn't enough to dismiss this argument, it also commits the *Appeal to Nature* fallacy. We covered this fallacy in chapter three and the conclusion remains the same here: because something is natural (i.e. it exists in nature) that does not justify it or make it good. To suggest otherwise is to take an illogical and dishonest leap. Ultimately, this popular argument commits multiple logical fallacies, thus it completely fails to justify homosexuality.

**Appropriate Response:** Natural human sexual intercourse is between a male and a female, and it's an undeniable fact that the natural purpose of sex is procreation. Procreation is impossible through homosexuality. It's an obvious and undeniable fact that male and female genitalia are specifically designed to be exclusively compatible with one another. In other words, males and females are sexually complementary by nature. Homosexuality violates this natural design and is therefore clearly unnatural. This is proven by the impossibility of procreation (the natural purpose of sex) coupled with the abundance of negative physical, mental, and emotional damage homosexuality causes. Therefore, you simply cannot look to animal behavior, where morality is nonexistent, to attempt to justify human behavior; especially when that behavior has been proven to be unnatural and immoral.

**10. "I'm actually quite offended."**
*Logical Fallacy Committed: Appeal to Emotion*—attempting to elicit an emotional response to justify one's position, especially when lacking any factual evidence.

**Note:** This is actually a tricky one. We live in a hypersensitive, politically correct driven society that says: "If it's offensive, or could possibly be offensive, then you're not allowed to say it." This ridiculous notion is counterintuitive because just about everything these days is considered offensive, which means no one would be allowed to say much of anything. Nevertheless, people have actually adopted this mindset and some skeptics have begun to use this as a tactic to censor Christians. While it is certainly not our objective to be offensive, some people will be offended by the truth even if we share it in a loving and respectful way. This does not mean the solution is to stop sharing the truth. There's a difference between being offended by a *person*, which is the implication here, and being offended by the *truth*, which is the reality. Anyone who is offended by the truth is living outside the truth, but instead of acknowledging that and making a positive change, the complacent sometimes respond with "I'm offended." Why? Because they know the natural response is an instinctive apology and a promise to not repeat the "offense." In this case, the desired response is, "I am so sorry. I didn't mean to offend you. I won't bring this up anymore, okay?" This is a clever, albeit dishonest way to silence someone in order to continue sinning in peace. Keep this in mind and remember our primary objective is to be led by the Spirit to share the truth with love and respect. In so doing the Spirit will assist us in being inoffensive in our approach and will also alert us when someone claims to be offended as a tactic to avoid the truth.

**Appropriate Response:** If you are offended by the truth, I cannot help that. Jesus is the truth. He offended people with the truth all the time but He never changed His message to appease the hearer; He challenged the hearer to change and accept the truth. Likewise, it is not my intention to offend you but rather to challenge you to accept the truth about homosexuality.

# Conclusion

Did any of these rebuttals actually disprove the conclusions we've reached? Not at all. In fact, they were all as irrational and illogical as the popular pro-homosexual arguments we examined in chapters two and three. So let's summarize our progress thus far. We've considered three answers to the question "Is homosexuality sinful?" Here's what we've established:

- "I don't know" is an irresponsible and unacceptable response.
- "No" is illogical and irrational considering all the fallacious arguments that fail to substantiate it.
- "Yes," is both logical and rational considering the abundance of evidence that substantiates it.

We even examined ten popular rebuttals from "homosexuals" and advocates and established why they all failed to contradict our conclusion. The verdict is in. Whatever is immoral is sinful. Thus, whether we examine homosexuality from a biblical or natural standpoint, the result remains the same: homosexuality is sinful/immoral.

There are honest, rational "homosexuals" and advocates who will accept this fact and subsequently change their pro-homosexual lifestyle and worldview. This is the optimal result. Others, as we have seen, will refuse to concede that homosexuality is sinful/immoral. This doesn't change the facts. Anyone who rejects both logical arguments and the overwhelming amount of supporting evidence is either confused or dishonest.

To the Christians who accept the truth that homosexuality is sinful, you now know how to present your position rationally and logically. You also know how to respond to rebuttals without backtracking or being manipulated. However, beware of those who merely want to argue. Sometimes, no matter how much sense you make, some people will refuse to accept the truth because they've hardened their hearts. They want to believe homosexuality isn't sinful so much that they will deny everything that proves otherwise. Jesus Christ himself could come down from heaven and tell them "Homosexuality is sinful," and they still wouldn't believe it. Do not be discouraged by this or resort to arguing. It's not that these hard-hearted individuals don't *know* the truth, or don't *understand* the truth; they simply refuse to *accept* the truth.

This is the epitome of self-deception. Still, don't give up on them. Instead of wasting your time and energy on pointless arguments, you can invest that time and energy in praying for those individuals and showing them the love of Christ through your lifestyle. You never know what the future holds. God may use something you've said or done to penetrate their hearts and you might witness a miraculous change in them one day.

# 5

## Can a "Homosexual" Go to Heaven?

Now that we've established that homosexuality is indeed sinful, the questions that immediately follow concern the spiritual and eternal ramifications of homosexuality. Does God hate "homosexuals"? Do all "homosexuals" go to hell? Isn't God a God of forgiveness? What about "homosexuals" who are really good people? What about "homosexuals" who are Christians and truly love God? What about people who struggle with homosexuality but can't seem to break free of the lifestyle? What happens to them?

These are all valid questions that deserve answers, particularly for those of us who have "homosexual" loved ones, and even more so for those who identify as "homosexuals." For the latter it's not, "What happens to *them*?" but rather, "What happens to *me*?" The underlying theme to all of these inquiries can be summed up in one critical question: "Can a 'homosexual' go to heaven?" The consensus is divided. There are Christians who say, "No, 'homosexuals' can't go to heaven," and then there are Christians who say, "Yes, 'homosexuals' can go to heaven." So who is right?

We can't possibly answer the question about "homosexuals" without first establishing how anyone gets to heaven. Jesus made the answer clear for us in the Bible. In John 14:6, Jesus said, "I am the way and the truth and the life. No one comes to the Father except through me." In fact, the reason God sent Jesus to earth was for Him to save mankind from sin and forge the way back to God the Father. So the answer to how anyone gets to heaven is quite simply through Jesus Christ. This means we acknowledge Christ suffered and died to save us, and in doing so, He has offered us the free gift of salvation. In accepting this gift, one declares Jesus Christ is their Lord and Savior. They repent for their sins, they ask Christ to come into their heart and wash them clean. From that moment on they vow to live a Godly lifestyle in total submission to Jesus. It is those who are followers of Christ, the true Christians, who go to heaven. However, as I've said before, there are millions of people who claim to be Christians but are not Christians at all. So can a "homosexual" be a Christian? If so, how can we be certain that those individuals are truly Christians and will go to heaven, as opposed to those who only claim to be Christians but are actually sinners? Let's consider a list of some Christian characteristics as expressed in the Bible to make the distinction clear.

## Christian Characteristics

### Jesus Is Our *Lord* and Savior
It's amazing to me how often people recite: "Jesus is my Lord and Savior," but only acknowledge the Savior aspect of Christ while totally ignoring the Lord aspect. In other words, they happily acknowledge Christ saved them from sin and death,

but they totally disregard the part where Christ is now in full control of their lives. This is a grave mistake. Christ's position in our lives is not something we can partially accept; it's something we must fully accept. If Christ is truly the Lord of your life, then you are no longer in control. This means you don't obey the urges of your sinful nature the way you did before you accepted Christ. Now that Christ is in your heart, you are filled with the Spirit, you are led by the Spirit, and you refuse to indulge your sinful nature any longer. That's what it means for Christ to be your Lord. It is not to say that we become robots, but we are simply committed to obeying Christ at all times in every area of our lives. The Bible tells us plainly, "You are not your own; you were purchased at a price" (1 Corinthians 6:19–20). Christians recognize we do not belong to ourselves; we belong to God. Since we belong to God, He has control over our lives—we don't. Therefore, we are totally submitted to Christ and keep His commands regardless of how we feel, or what we think. Anyone who refuses to allow Christ to take His rightful leadership role as Lord of his or her life is not a Christian.

## We Don't Practice Sin

Despite the fact that many Christians claim they are still sinners and make false statements such as, "We all can't help but sin every day," the truth is Christians do not practice sin. That is not to say we are perfect and never sin, but remaining perfectly sinless is indeed the goal we constantly strive for. We are distinguished from those who practice sin because when we sin we are immediately convicted. It hurts to disobey God, and it affects us in such a powerfully negative way that we can't help but to repent, adjust our lives, and reconcile ourselves to God. The longer we are Christians, the closer we become to God, and the less we sin. We are not on a merry-go-round or a rollercoaster; we are on a continuous path that leads towards righteousness and away from sin. We were not created to be sinful creatures, and Christ did not die for our sins so that we could in turn embrace sinfulness and practice it. Christians practice righteousness and godliness, not sinfulness. In fact, Galatians 5:24 makes this clear: "Those who belong to Christ Jesus have crucified the sinful nature with its passions and desires." The antithesis of this Scripture is that those who continue to obey their sinful nature and feed its passions and desires do *not* belong to Christ. To store sin in one's heart and have Jesus in one's heart are two conflicting realities. It's either one or the other because light and darkness cannot dwell in the same place at the same time. We find the distinction between Christians and sinners made quite clearly in 1 John 2:4–6, which says, "The man who says, 'I know [Jesus]' but does not do what he commands is a liar, and the truth is not in him. But if anyone obeys his word, God's love is truly made complete in him. This is how we know we are in him: Whoever claims to live in him must walk as Jesus did." Jesus led a sinless life, so if we are in Christ and He is in us, we must strive to live sinless lives as well. Those who claim to be Christians yet live sinful lives are by definition sinners, not Christians.

## We Believe the Bible is the Inerrant Word of God

Christians understand the Bible is not only the Word of God, but the Word of God is inerrant. The logic is simple:

1. God is inerrant.
2. The Bible is the Word of God
3. Therefore, the Bible is inerrant.

This means because God cannot lie, and His Word is truth, nothing in it is false. This truth is repeatedly expressed in the Bible:

> "For the word of the Lord is right and true"
> (Psalm 33:4).

"Every word of God is flawless" (Proverbs 30:5).

"All Scripture is God-breathed and is useful for teaching, rebuking, correcting and training in righteousness, so that the man of God may be thoroughly equipped for every good work" (2 Timothy 3:16-17).

"For the word of God is living and active. Sharper than any double-edged sword, it penetrates even to dividing soul and spirit, joints and marrow; it judges the thoughts and attitudes of the heart" (Hebrews 4:12).

Now, we do not believe these bold claims the Bible makes for itself simply because it's in the Bible; that would be circular reasoning. We believe these bold claims because the Bible repeatedly proves these claims to be true. The proof is in the evidence: fulfilled prophesy, archeology, science, historicity, and the evidence of our personal experience with God through His Word all point directly to the fact that the Word of God is inerrant. Despite the fact that God used men to write the Bible, and men copied the original manuscripts of the Bible, we know God was involved in the process. God ensured His Holy Word was preserved for us because we desperately need it. Therefore, we stand on God's Word, we study God's Word, and we live by God's Word. This is a critical Christian characteristic because I've heard professing Christians say, "I don't believe the Bible is inerrant," in order to justify sin. In fact, Tom, the young "homosexual" I referenced earlier, told me this after I proved the Bible clearly refutes his claim that homosexuality is not sin. He thought denying the inerrancy of God's Word would somehow support his claim but it doesn't. Can someone truly be a Christian and believe God's word is filled with errors? What's more, how can someone who doubts the truth of God's Word determine which biblical commands are actually from God and which one's aren't? For example, Tom said he believes fornication and adultery are sinful even for "homosexuals", so I asked him how he could possibly believe that. By what power or knowledge can he decide fornication and adultery are indeed sinful, but homosexuality isn't because it is one of the errors made in God's Word? Of course he was unable to provide me with an answer, because there isn't one that makes any sense. Based on his irrational thinking, any professing Christian could present a counterargument that fornication or adultery are actually not sinful because *those* are errors in God's Word. This picking and choosing which Scriptures to follow and which ones to ignore based on one's own sinful proclivities is precisely why people claim Christians are hypocrites. The fact, however, is Christians are not hypocrites, and hypocrites are not Christians. Therefore, anyone who denies the inerrancy of God's Word in an effort to rationalize his or her sinful proclivities is simply not a Christian.

### We Obey Proverbs 3:5

We trust in the Lord wholeheartedly like this Scripture commands us, regardless if we fully understand His commands or not. We do not lean to our own understanding because we know we are fallible, while God is infallible. We know God leads us on the paths we would never find on our own, so we gladly get out of the proverbial driver's seat and move to the passenger's seat so Jesus can control where we go. By contrast, the ones who don't trust God wholeheartedly, the ones who are always questioning God's commandments and refusing to follow them until they fully understand them, the ones who trust their feelings, desires, and knowledge above God, all violate this command and exclude themselves from being a Christian by definition.

**We Love God with all Our Heart, Soul, Mind, and Strength**
This means we put God first in our lives, we love Him with the whole of our being, and we love Him more than anything and anyone else. Anything and anyone else includes sin, sex, and significant others. If your significant other is more important to you than God is, then you are completely out of order. People who claim to be Christians often profess their love for God but rarely understand how God determines who loves Him and who doesn't. It's not at all what we *say*; it's what we *do* that proves our love for God. Jesus said:

> If you love me, you will obey what I command . . . Whoever has my commands and obeys them, he is the one who loves me . . . If anyone loves me, he will obey my teaching. My father will love him, and we will come to him and make our home with him. He who does not love me will not obey my teaching (John 14:15, 21, 23–24).

Notice two things: first the qualifier "if" in the statement, "*If* you love me." That's a clear indication that it's not about words. So saying, "I love God," or, "I'm a Christian," a million times every day means absolutely nothing. Secondly, notice how often Jesus repeated how love for Him is demonstrated: through *obedience*. Those who obey His word don't have to say anything because they prove their love for God by how they live. Likewise, those who disobey God's Word don't have to say anything because they prove they don't love God by how they live. This means we not only study the Bible in order to know God's commands in order to follow them, but we don't pick and choose which Scriptures we'll follow. Christians are dedicated to obeying God's commandments; sinners are dedicated to disobeying God's commandments.

One simply cannot be dedicated to disobeying God and be a Christian.

## We Love Our Neighbors as Ourselves

This means we treat others the way we would want to be treated. In proving our love for our neighbors, we do not ignore their sinful behavior but try to save them from their sinful behavior; and we certainly don't engage in sinful behavior with them. We do not simply care about saving our own souls and then remain quiet so we don't offend anyone by telling them the truth. We don't live our lives without concern for the souls of others. We are as concerned about their well being and eternal destination as we are about our own. Thus, we spend our lives shining the light of Christ and helping others out of darkness as we are led by the Holy Spirit. That's the sign of a true Christian—we look out for one another. Proverbs 27:17 says, "As iron sharpens iron, so one man sharpens another." We are in this race together, and we are all dedicated to helping one another be victorious in Christ. Those who are only concerned about their own salvation and refuse to help save the lost are working *against* Christ not *for* Christ. In addition, those who engage in sinful practices like homosexuality, even if they believe it's an act of love, are violating this Scripture; they are proving by their actions that they are sinners not Christians.

# True Christianity

What I've listed here are a few key characteristics that collectively establish the definition of a Christian. One can't take a few things from each, or choose a couple and ignore the rest and still be a Christian, and yet that is what many people believe. I continue to hear this oxymoronic term "liberal Christian."

These are professing Christians who try to modify God's Word and position themselves on the wrong side of controversial issues. I encouraged Christians to abstain from reading and watching illicit content like the popular *Fifty Shades of Grey.* I condemned the deplorable violence against women under Islamic Sharia Law. I've challenged people to stop endorsing homosexuality and help people overcome homosexuality. In every one of these instances I've been chastised repeatedly by "liberal Christians" who either approve of sinfulness or insist it's hateful to speak against sinfulness. I've actually had a "liberal Christian" encourage me to forsake my vow of celibacy and start having sex because "God understands." He had premarital sex and wound up getting married. I refuse to have premarital sex and I've obviously yet to marry. So in his mind I should just give in and have sex to get a wife. He attempted to justify this by claiming we all sin every day, and God will forgive us anyway, so it's not that big of a deal. In his mind, it's worth sinning to get something you want; in my mind, if it takes sin to get it, then I don't want it.

This liberal concept that it's acceptable to play Christian when it's convenient, but otherwise play sinner, is absurd. The fact is there is no such thing as a "liberal Christian." Anyone who identifies as a "liberal Christian" is a sinner who is lying to himself or herself. There is also no such thing as customized Christianity. We can't pick and choose what we like and don't like about Christianity, what we agree with and disagree with, which of God's commands we'll follow and won't follow, and still call that Christianity. That's not Christianity. Likewise, there is no such thing as a "practicing gay Christian."

Now, this is where we must be clear on our definitions. Remember that our definition of *"homosexual"/"gay"/ "lesbian" is an individual who finds himself or herself sexually attracted to members of the same gender.* In other words: someone who experiences SSA. Based on this definition, a "gay Christian" is a person who experiences SSA but models their life after Jesus Christ and the Gospel and thus abstains from homosexuality and all sexual sinfulness. A "practicing gay Christian," however, is *an individual whose lifestyle involves the willful engagement in erotic behavior with members of the same gender* but affirms Christianity. This is tantamount to a "sinner Christian," which is clearly self-contradictory. There is no such thing as an "adulterous Christian," "a promiscuous Christian," an "incestuous Christian," a "pedophile Christian," etc., so there cannot possibly be such thing as a "practicing homosexual Christian." Jesus Christ Himself was celibate, so a Christian modeling one's life after Christ cannot reconcile any sexually immoral lifestyle with our perfect primary example for life. None of Christ's teachings, and nowhere in the whole of Scripture for that matter, is homosexuality deemed moral or acceptable in any way. It is important to reiterate this point because there are individuals who believe it is possible to be a "gay Christian," and by their definition they mean a "practicing gay Christian." This is a terrible mistake. The Scripture is crystal clear on this issue. A Christian who experiences SSA, but consistently denies those feelings and pleases God in their thoughts, speech, and actions will indeed go to heaven. An individual who experiences SSA and indulges in homosexuality cannot please God even if they've convinced themselves and everyone else they are a Christian. God knows the difference: the distinction is clear and there is no gray area or compromising to rationalize sinfulness.

Now if this offends you or upsets you, please remember you don't have to be a Christian. Again, no one is forcing you to do anything. However, do remember what is at stake. We've learned Christ is the only way to God. Christians are the only ones who go to heaven because Christians are children of God and co-heirs with Christ. If you insist on rejecting Christianity and continuing to live the life of a sinner, or straddling the fence between Christianity and sin, then you've made your position quite clear. Jesus is not your Lord, you choose to continue practicing sin, you choose to continue violating Proverbs 3:5, you do not love God with all your heart, soul, mind and strength, and you do not love your neighbor as yourself, because if you did, you wouldn't be sinning with your neighbor or showing others how to live a sinful life. This is the path to destruction.

Now, God doesn't send these individuals to hell as many claim. Those who fit into this category have chosen to go to hell themselves by not choosing to obey God. It is astonishing how many times in the Bible God pleads with us by saying, "Obey my commands." He says it time and time again in Scripture, but like the perfect gentleman that He is, He doesn't force us to do anything. He's presented the solution, He's urged us repeatedly to accept the solution, but He has left the decision to us. Those who reject the solution are left with the problem and will suffer the consequences of their decision.

So how does this apply to homosexuality? Remember homosexuality is a behavior; we defined homosexuality as "erotic behavior with members of the same gender." We've determined this behavior is sinful, and therefore anyone who practices this behavior is a sinner, not a Christian. Again this is not limited to "homosexuals." There are "straight" people who choose to indulge in homosexuality, and this behavior is prohibited for them as well. So now the question is, is it possible to identify as a "homosexual" and not indulge in homosexuality? The answer is: absolutely, although, again I don't recommend anyone self-identify according to their sexuality, especially not sinful sexualities. Nevertheless, there are countless "ex-homosexuals" who have explained their transition out of the "homosexual" lifestyle, and it is indeed possible to refrain from "homosexual" activity despite experiencing same-sex attraction. Like drug addicts who are clean and sober still refer to themselves as addicts, though they are doing everything in their power to abandon that destructive lifestyle forever, a person can say, "I once identified myself as a homosexual, but now I identify myself as a Christian. I now refuse to indulge in homosexuality or even entertain impure thoughts because I love the Lord with all my heart, soul, mind, and strength. I have changed from the lifestyle of a sinner to the lifestyle of a Christian, and I'm never turning back." Now I'm well aware it takes much more than a positive declaration to transition out of the "homosexual" lifestyle (which we will discuss in more detail later), but the point remains valid.

# Conclusion

*Can a "homosexual" go to heaven?* is a critical question. The answer is a resounding *yes*. They simply must be a *practicing Christian,* not a *practicing "homosexual."* If a person who identifies as "gay" truly gives their life to Christ, they will obey God's Word and refrain from living a "homosexual" lifestyle. Whether they struggle with "homosexual" thoughts and urges for the rest of their lives (as I continue to struggle with sexual thoughts and urges despite the fact that I refuse to act on them), or they join the countless others who transition completely out of the "homosexual" lifestyle and no longer experience SSA, as long as Jesus Christ is the center of their lives and they are wholeheartedly devoted to serving Him, then they will go to heaven. This is pivotal because many Christians forget about the transition and make blanket statements like, "All 'gays' are going to hell." This is not only false; it's ignorant and insensitive. No one who has ever lived a sinful lifestyle was instantly freed forever of all their sinful *urges* upon deciding to turn their life over to Christ. Yes, they were instantly saved once they accepted Christ into their hearts and repented of their sins, but then it took time to learn how to maintain a Christian lifestyle by denying sinful urges instead of continuing to live the life of a sinner by giving in to them. The same thing holds true for "homosexuals." Because someone identifies as "gay" doesn't mean they are a "practicing homosexual," nor does that mean they are going to hell. When "gay" people truly dedicate their lives to Christ, they learn to stop identifying themselves as "gay," and they start identifying as a new creation is Christ Jesus. Even if their struggle with SSA continues and they never actually act on those attractions, or even entertain sexual thoughts out of reverence for Christ. Remember that in 1 Corinthians 6:9 the Apostle Paul warned that homosexual offenders would not inherit the kingdom of heaven, but he didn't stop there. In verse eleven he adds some spectacular and inspiring news: "That is what some of you *were*. But you were washed, you were sanctified, you were justified in the name of the Lord Jesus Christ and by the Holy Spirit of our God." Those in this category, who have renounced their submission to homosexuality and have become wholeheartedly submitted to Christ, will indeed go to heaven.

# 6

# What About Loving Committed "Gay" Relationships?

This question is either asked with the ulterior motive of attempting to rationalize "good 'homosexual' relationships," or the motive of genuinely seeking understanding. I will address both by responding briefly to the former and then dedicating the bulk of this chapter to the latter. One of the more popular proponents of the position that all same-sex relationships are not sinful is a young man named Matthew Vines. Matthew is a "homosexual," a professing Christian, and an "LGBT" activist. He is the president and founder of The Reformation Project, an organization solely dedicated to changing the Christian position on homosexuality. Of course, any Christian who has honestly read the Bible knows it is impossible to merge Christianity with homosexuality without distorting or ignoring the Scripture. This is precisely what Matthew resorts to in an effort to justify homosexuality, and sadly he has spread his deception to untold others. Matthew essentially claims homosexuality isn't a sin, and

God only condemns lust-driven homosexuality. The trouble is Matthew's arguments to legitimize this bold claim are wrought with error, contradiction, and logical fallacies. When presenting his case, Matthew excels at manipulating his audience by distorting Scripture, misrepresenting facts, appealing to emotion, and presenting false dilemmas. Let's examine a few excerpts from his hour-long presentation *The Gay Debate: The Bible and Homosexuality.*[35]

**"The Bible never directly addresses sexual orientation."**
Firstly, we must not forget why this assertion is absurd. Remember that "sexual orientation" doesn't exist. It is a figment of the imagination; a concept invented in an effort to legitimize sexual immorality. Given this, it is perfectly clear why the Bible never addresses "sexual orientation." It isn't real! Thus, Matthew's assertion is clearly biased, manipulative, and holds absolutely no weight. Moreover, even if we are among the millions who actually believe "sexual orientation" is real and that we all have one, this argument still fails. What Matthew infers here is the biblical condemnation of homosexuality can't possibly apply to anyone with a "homosexual orientation" because the Bible fails to even address "sexual orientation." Matthew assumes this means the biblical condemnation of homosexuality is specifically limited to the lustful, but this is illogical. The absence of "sexual orientation" in Scripture does not mean everyone with a "homosexual orientation" is exempt from condemnation. On the contrary, the Scripture is clear: all "homosexual" *behavior* is prohibited for *everyone* regardless of his or her "sexual orientation." The Bible clearly limits sex to within the confines of marriage between a man and a woman, and any sexual activity outside of those limits is sinful. God's command doesn't magically change for those who invoke a "homosexual orientation" as Matthew suggests, simply because the concept isn't addressed in the Bible. Keep in mind God

doesn't identify us by our sexuality anyway, so it wouldn't make any sense for "sexual orientation" to be included in the Bible. Further, remember that pedophiles have already begun to insist if there's such a thing as a "sexual orientation," then their "sexual orientation" points toward young children, and they shouldn't be prevented from having loving committed relationships either. So following Matthew's "logic," a pedophile could argue that because the Bible doesn't directly address "sexual orientation," God approves of pedophilia as long as it's a loving and committed relationship. This clearly is totally erroneous reasoning.

**"[The Bible] certainly does not condemn loving committed same-sex relationships . . . "**
This argument fails immediately because the Bible certainly does not *approve* of "loving committed same-sex relationships." Moreover, why would the Bible specifically condemn "loving committed same-sex relationships" when it repeatedly condemns homosexuality? If homosexuality is sinful, which we've already established it is, then all "homosexual" *behavior* and *relationships* built on that *behavior* are sinful. Again, if we follow Matthew's "logic," one could argue the Bible doesn't condemn loving committed incestuous, adulterous, or polyamorous relationships, but this obviously fails because the Bible condemns incest, adultery, and polyamory. Any relationship based on sinful behavior is sinful, plain and simple.

**" . . . nor is there any call to lifelong celibacy for gay people."**
Matthew is vehemently opposed to lifelong celibacy, which brings his motives into question. If his goal is to twist Scripture to rationalize having sex, then he has placed sexual immorality before God and is therefore an idolater. Further, we cannot forget that the concept of a distinction between "gay people" and "straight people" is a modern concept that

is contrary to how God identifies us. This is why the Bible doesn't address "gay people" *at all*, let alone prescribe life-long celibacy for them. Again, the Bible sets the standard for good and right *behavior* for *everyone* and then condemns anything outside of it. In an effort to avoid this undeniable fact, Matthew repeats his faulty formula: "The Bible doesn't say X, so therefore God must approve of X." As we've seen, this is entirely false. Every willing and eligible person has the option to participate in God's marriage, and anyone unwilling and/or ineligible is called to remain sexually pure. This is a universal standard. So as I desired to be married, have sex, and have children from an early age, because I have not fallen in love with anyone I wish to marry, I must remain sexually pure even if I never fall in love. This is what I have done and will continue to do indefinitely because it is God's command. If Matthew is truly a Christian, he is obligated to follow the same command, even though his struggle is different.

**"But the Bible does explicitly reject forced loneliness as God's will for human beings."**
This claim is yet another distortion of Scripture, and frankly a lie. The concept of "forced loneliness" is based on Matthew's misinterpretation of Genesis 2:18 when God said of Adam, "It is not good for the man to be alone." Notice who God referred to when He said, "the man"? He referred specifically to Adam. He didn't say, "It is not good for all men to be alone." Matthew has ignored this fact. Further, there is a difference between being alone and being lonely. In Matthew's misinter-pretation, Adam was lonely, and God said loneliness wasn't good, which means it's wrong to force someone to be lonely. Therefore, God approves loving committed same-sex rela-tionships because the alternative is "forced loneliness." This couldn't be more illogical. There is obviously a fundamental distinction between the first and only human on the planet earth, and a "gay" person in today's society who professes

Christianity and has the desire to get married and have "gay" sex. Adam's divine purpose was to populate the earth, and for that he needed a suitable helper, which was a woman. Matthew Vines' purpose is not to populate the earth, and so he cannot compare himself to Adam or declare the Bible prohibits "forced loneliness" in an effort to rationalize homosexuality. This assertion fails completely because it is a lie.

**"If the remedy against sexual sin for straight Christians is marriage, why should the remedy for gay Christians not be the same?"**
This is another distortion of Scripture. Here Matthew is referencing the Apostle Paul's instruction to the unmarried in 1 Corinthians 7:9, which says, "But if they cannot control themselves, they should marry, for it is better to marry than to burn with passion." Matthew, by his own admission, doesn't fit into this category. In his presentation he said he's never been in a relationship and has always believed in abstinence until marriage. This proves that he's not burning with passion but has self-control. Moreover, he presumes the remedy for sexual sin is marriage, which is false. The remedy for sexual sin, and *all* sin, is Jesus Christ. So this assertion also fails because it is fallacious.

**"I love God. And I love Jesus. I really do. But that doesn't mean that I need to hate myself, or somehow wallow in self-pity, misery, and loathing for the rest of my life. That's not what God created me to do."**
This is classic Matthew Vines. Here he commits what's called the *Appeal to Emotion* fallacy, which is attempting to elicit an emotional response to justify one's position, especially when lacking any factual evidence. In addition, he commits the *Black and White* fallacy, which is to present two alternatives as the only possibilities, when in truth more possibilities exist. Let's deal with his profession of love first. We've discussed how

God measures love, and that is through the keeping of His commandments. Matthew's fundamental problem is he's removed God's Word from the supreme position in his life, replaced it with his sexuality, and then attempted to alter God's word to fit his sexuality. God's commands stand alone. We either agree with them or we don't. We either wholeheartedly obey them or we don't. Our decisions prove whether we love God or not. Matthew's following statements are obviously true albeit misleading. His desire is to manipulate an emotional response that says, "Oh that's horrible. Nobody deserves to suffer like that. Maybe loving committed 'gay' relationships aren't sinful after all." Do not fall into this trap. First of all, *nobody* was created to hate themselves, and "wallow in self-pity, misery, and loathing" for the rest of their lives. Secondly, to allege this is the sole consequence of adhering to God's Word is absurd and manipulative. The multitudes of Christians, who have battled SSA their entire lives but maintain their celibacy, can attest to the fact that Christians are blessed of God. Christians have a peace that passes understanding and a joy that's unspeakable because our identities aren't built on our sexuality, but on Christ who lives within us. If Matthew isn't experiencing these fruits of Christianity, then he's ignoring a much larger problem while perpetrating his misrepresentation of reality. By creating this false dilemma, Matthew has purposely disregarded the real possibility of joining countless others in overcoming SSA. He's also disregarded the real possibility of living a peaceful and fulfilling life in honoring God through lifelong celibacy like the Apostle Paul recommended and which I can personally attest to.

It's fascinating to me how Matthew began by claiming Jesus warned of false teachers in an effort to sway his audience, and then proceeded with an hour-long dissertation of false teaching. Then, in the entire course of his speech, he offered *no proof whatsoever* that his claims are actually true. The fact is God is all-knowing, which means if there was indeed an exception for loving committed same-sex relationships, God would have made that perfectly clear in His Word. He didn't—a fact that Matthew totally ignores. He has failed to construct a proper logical argument to prove his bold conclusions, and consequently, many biblical scholars have responded to Matthew and dismantled his entire argument. Matthew, who authored a book entitled *God and the Gay Christian: The Biblical Case in Support of Same-Sex Relationships,* engaged in a debate with Dr. Michael Brown, author of *Can You Be Gay and Christian?: Responding With Love and Truth to Questions About Homosexuality.* Matthew was soundly defeated by Dr. Brown, and yet, instead of altering his position in light of the truth, he continues down the path of deception. In fact, since losing that debate, despite continuous offers, Matthew refuses to debate anyone else who has proven his book to be as fallacious as his presentation. The reason is obvious: Matthew Vines *wants* God to approve of homosexuality, but he knows he cannot prove that God actually *approves* of homosexuality. Yet he continues to try to make the Bible say what it doesn't say. As a general rule, any time it takes that much energy, effort, and explanation to try to make the Bible say something other than what it actually says, that interpretation is wrong. I pray Matthew Vines comes to this conclusion and gives God his whole heart in order to fulfill his divine purpose in life. If Matthew Vines is truly a Christian, he is well aware our primary objective beyond loving God and our neighbors is to share the gospel of Jesus Christ. Clearly Matthew's sole objective is to promote homosexuality in the church. This is unfortunate because he's already amassed a significant following with his "progressive" position. Instead of leading people away from God through deception, I believe Matthew could lead scores of people to God through the truth, if he only changed his focus from promoting homosexuality to promoting God. So be careful, my brothers and sisters. Do not be swayed by false doctrines wrapped in a package that grips your heart. Emotions don't alter God's Word.

# Genuine Seekers

Now for those who are genuinely seeking to understand *why* same-sex relationships based on love and commitment are sinful even though they appear to be good, let's examine this closer. We'll begin with a short list of fundamental principles we must keep in mind as we proceed. In demystifying homosexuality more questions will most likely arise, and recalling these principles will often answer those questions.

### 5 Fundamental Principles of Life
1. God is perfect and the highest form of good.
2. Everything God creates flows from His goodness and is therefore good.
3. Everything God creates has a divine purpose, and the fulfillment of that purpose is also good.
4. Anything that violates the goodness and purpose of God's creations is sinful.
5. Justice is good, it is the rightful response to evil, and it demands the atonement and eradication of all evil.

When we take the logical conclusions we've reached thus far concerning the sinfulness of homosexuality and run them against these five principles, it becomes quite clear why homosexuality violates God's Moral Law without exception. However, we won't stop there. Let's continue down this path by examining all the critical elements involved: mankind, love, marriage, sex, and family. We will examine each of these from God's perspective and from the pro-homosexual perspective, and then we will compare and contrast the two.

Please note: pro-homosexual refers to practicing "homosexuals" as well as advocates, which again are *individuals who are not "homosexual" themselves, but passionately promote and defend homosexuality.*

# Mankind

Mankind is the basest common element in the "homosexual" equation and is comprised of both man and woman. According to the fundamental principles we've listed, mankind was good at the point of creation, and both man and woman retain a specific purpose for which they were created. Let's examine mankind from both perspectives.

## ACCORDING TO GOD

*Definition of Mankind*
According to God, mankind is defined as the only beings in all existence that were created as a reflection of God. "God created man in His own image, in the image of God He created him; male and female He created them" (Genesis 1:27). Male and female were made in God's image and in His likeness, a characteristic that is entirely unique to humans. Male and female are themselves unique and complementary genders, each with specific roles to play in society, primarily husband and father for the male, and wife and mother for the female.

*Purpose of Mankind*
Mankind was created out of love to be loved and to love. The first priority is a loving relationship with God and second is to be in loving relationships with one another. To accomplish this, Adam and Eve, the first male and female, were given a specific purpose in Genesis 1:28: "God blessed them and said

to them, 'Be fruitful and increase in number; fill the earth and subdue it. Rule over the fish of the sea and the birds of the air and over every living creature that moves on the ground.'"

Later, Jesus summed up mankind's purpose in two simple commands. In Matthew 22:37–39 he says, "'Love the Lord your God with all your heart and with all your soul and with all your mind.' This is the first and greatest commandment. And the second is like it: 'Love your neighbor as yourself.'" This applies to everyone, men and women, the single and the married. In accordance with this, man and woman, each being distinct from the other, have specific purposes to fulfill. What is the purpose of man? To work, to protect his loved ones, to provide for his loved ones, and to be Christ-like, especially in the two most important roles of husband and father. What is the purpose of woman? To be Christ-like especially in the two most important roles of wife and mother, and to help man fulfill his purpose. Now many women take this as a negative, but it is an extreme positive. The Bible makes it abundantly clear that man needs help. It also makes it abundantly clear that woman is the only creation in all existence suitable for the task. God blessed women to be phenomenal multitaskers: they are fully capable of fulfilling their own purpose while simultaneously aiding man in fulfilling his purpose. A man simply cannot successfully fulfill his purpose as a husband and father without his wife, and vice versa. So in the end, man's purpose is fulfilled through Christ and with the help of his suitable partner, and woman's purpose is fulfilled through Christ and in the helping of man, her suitable partner. Moreover, to fulfill God's command of filling the earth, man surely cannot do so on his own, nor can woman do so on her own. Man needs woman's help, and woman needs man's help. This is the foundation of the loving, beneficial, and exclusive relationship known as marriage, which is good because God created it. It is through marriage that God's will is done for man and woman.

## ACCORDING TO PRO-HOMOSEXUALS

*Definition of Mankind*

According to pro-homosexuals, mankind is defined as a race of human beings, each identified by a chosen gender, which may or may not conflict with their biological sex. In the minds of pro-homosexuals, sexes (male and female) exist, but a distinction is made between sex and gender, and it is asserted sex does not determine gender. Gender is redefined as the concept each individual has of his or herself and includes male, female, both male and female, or neither male nor female along with many other invented gender types. As such, this concept could align or conflict with one's sex. Of course, this assertion immediately raises questions because it seems to stand in direct conflict with "LGBT" ideology, which asserts "sexual orientation" is determined, not chosen. In other words, "gays" and "lesbians" are "born that way," but despite how everyone is born, people can choose their own gender. How can it be impossible to not choose a "sexual orientation," but be possible to choose a gender? It's interesting that pro-homosexuals have looked to genetics in an effort to prove people are born "homosexual", and yet they ignore the fact that regardless of any surgeries and hormones an individual might take in an effort to change sexes, their genetic code never changes. Yet, are we to conclude that individuals like Bruce Jenner, who chose to adopt the female gender, literally become female? If so, what does Bruce Jenner's relationship to his children become? Surely it can't be father if he's no longer a man, and surely it couldn't be mother, because he did not give birth to them, nor is he capable of giving birth to a child. Further, if one day "Caitlyn Jenner" changes his mind (as many transsexuals do) and chooses to "return" to a male gender, does he become a male again? As ridiculous as this concept of "gender fluidity" is, pro-homosexuals believe that it is a reality. How these conclusions are reached, and how they shift from theory to "facts" remains a mystery. How these "facts" suddenly apply to all mankind is also unclear. What is clear is that blurring the line between the male and female genders causes all manner of complication and confusion. Now please understand I recognize these issues are real, they are serious, and they are complex. It is not my intention to trivialize this in any way. I'm merely pointing out the pro-homosexual view and the fact that a concept or idea is not necessarily factual, especially when all the factual evidence contradicts that concept or idea.

*Purpose of Mankind*
Pro-homosexuals believe mankind's purpose is to live in a world of freedom and equality where love has no limits or boundaries, and everyone can unashamedly be themselves without suffering persecution. It must be clearly understood that while love is the word almost exclusively used by pro-homosexuals to promote this ideology, the truth is love is secondary to sex. The concept of love without limits essentially means sex without limits. Sex in the "homosexual" community is the core component of love, but even in the absence of love, sex remains the priority. The issue is the world we currently live in does not fit the mold described here. This is why "homosexual" activists and "LGBT" organizations work tirelessly to change the world so it will fit their mold. If and when they are successful, there will no longer be "LGBT" communities within a larger community, there will be a single community that openly embraces and promotes the "homosexual" lifestyle, with no opposition. All churches and Christian organizations that oppose homosexuality will be eliminated, rendered silent, or converted to embrace and promote homosexuality. The laws will then change to allow all manners of sexual activity, everyone will be free to satisfy any and every sexual appetite with whomever they please as often as they please, and

the pro-homosexual purpose of mankind will finally be fulfilled through the indulgence of pleasure in place of the purpose of pleasing God. If this sounds familiar to you, it's because it is already happening.

**Comparing and Contrasting**
According to God, love is mankind's primary focus; sex is secondary and is bound by love in marriage. According to the pro-homosexuals, sex is mankind's primary focus; love is secondary and is bound by nothing. According to God, man is fundamentally distinct from woman, and the two species were created to reflect God and complement each other. According to pro-homosexuals, there is no such distinction between man and woman. One can change into the other at will (with the assistance of hormone therapy and destructive surgeries), and neither have a purpose unique to their sex. It is abundantly clear these are two totally contrary definitions. Both cannot be accurate, and since we've already established God is perfect, we can be assured His definition is correct as always. This obviously means the pro-homosexual definition of mankind is incorrect. Therefore, God's purpose for mankind prevails, and the pro-homosexual perception of mankind's purpose fails because it is inaccurate, it is outside of God's will, and it is inherently sinful.

# Love

Love is an essential and fundamental building block in good relationships of every category. Love must therefore be fully understood and properly expressed for two reasons: to ensure we enter the right relationships in life, and to ensure those relationships last and are fruitful for all parties involved.

## ACCORDING TO GOD

*Definition of Love*

God is the authority on love because God *is* love and love comes from God. 1 John 4:7–8 says, "Let us love one another, because love comes from God. Everyone who loves has been born of God and knows God. Whoever does not love does not know God, because God is love." This means mankind (the creation) cannot set the parameters for love or redefine love because we do not have the power to set the parameters for God or redefine Him. Only God is qualified to set the parameters for love and fully explain what love is because He is the source of love. We find God's definition of love all throughout His Word. Love is sacrifice, it is selfless, it is good, and it is pure.

> Love is patient, love is kind. It does not envy, it does not boast, it is not proud. It is not rude, it is not self-seeking, it is not easily angered, it keeps no record of wrongs. Love does not delight in evil but rejoices in the truth. It always protects, always trusts, always hopes, always perseveres. Love never fails (1 Corinthians 13:4–8).

All in all, love is a perfect reflection of God. Anything outside the parameters God has set for love is simply not love. Notice God's definition of love mentions nothing of intimacy or sex. The mistake people most commonly make is to assume love means sex or that sex means love, but this is a totally fallacious concept. Notice also that love is not proud. This contradicts the entire "homosexual" movement, which is built entirely on "gay *pride*," and being "out and *proud*." Love takes no pleasure in evil, which also contradicts the "homosexual" movement. If you've seen any recent footage or photos from "gay" pride parades, you've seen it literally is a celebration of evil. There is nudity, lewdness, and even anti-Christian displays at these events. Most often these anti-Christian displays feature nude "gay" and "lesbian" couples who are fixed to crosses. The couples then begin kissing each other to ridicule Christ in front of cheering crowds. Most recently I saw an image of a transgender "woman" who was made to look as though he'd been flogged. He was then fixed to a cross for all to see. Above the cross was a sign that said, "ENOUGH OF HOMOPHOBIA GLBT."

Equally disturbing is that in the past, children were brought to such parades and were exposed to these evils, but now children are actually made to participate in these events. Young boys are trained to dance sexually in front of cheering crowds while wearing little clothing. Yet people claim the "homosexual" movement is all about love? Not quite. Homosexuality, as we've come to learn, is impure and is evil in God's sight. Therefore, to love "homosexuals" is to help them out of homosexuality, not to encourage them in it or participate in it with them.

*Purpose of Love*
The purpose of love is ultimately to glorify God, but it is also the binding force of good pure relationships. God loved us first, and in reciprocating that love and extending God's love to one another, we are fulfilling our purpose and reflecting God in the process.

## ACCORDING TO PRO-HOMOSEXUALS

*Definition of Love*
As there are many types of relationships there are many types of love. One could love their mother, their friend, and their wife, but each one is loved in an entirely different way. It appears the primary focus of love in the "homosexual"

community is romantic love. In this case it could be defined as a feeling or emotion, which often results from the progression of physical attraction to erotic thoughts to erotic actions. Here love is sexual in the mind, in deed, or in both. Members of the "LGBT" community have argued love and sex are essentially the same and there is no distinction between the "homosexual" individual and their sexuality. So in other words, by having sex, "gays" and "lesbians" are naturally expressing love.

This concept was reaffirmed during a conversation I had with a practicing "lesbian" who was kind enough to open up to me about her lifestyle. She affirmed she was not born "gay," but specified she did not choose to be attracted to females. After recognizing this attraction, she described how her mind was overwhelmed with "homosexual" thoughts. At that point she reasoned she had two options: to remain single her entire life claiming to be "straight," but never being with a man, or to explore her desires and give herself the chance to fall in love. Curiously, she paused there to add, "because sex *is* a part of love," before concluding with, "I chose to live the way I was feeling, but I did not choose to feel that way." I found this quite strange because sex was not at all the topic of our conversation, but she saw fit to emphasize the perceived connection between love and sex while explaining the path she chose. Ironically, she unwittingly admitted her thoughts were not about falling in love, but were erotic and sexual in nature. By her own admission, in choosing to follow those "desires," she began having sexual encounters with other females not because she loved them, but because she had sexual feelings that she chose to act upon based on the *possibility* of falling in love in the future. This, of course, is totally contradictory to her claim that sex is a part of love. I kindly pointed this out by explaining that there are many types of love, but even in romantic love, sex is not an essential element: there are people who have sex all the time but are not in love, and there are couples (both married and unmarried) who are in love but don't have sex. To this she had no response. I believe it suddenly occurred to her that her concept of love was not love at all. To describe romantic love as she did (and as many others do), which is an intense uncontrollable sexual desire, is a mistake because that is not at all the definition of *love*. It is, however, the precise definition of *lust*.

*Purpose of Love*
I do not doubt the sincerity of the "homosexual" desire for love. I believe every human being needs to love and to be loved in this life, and just as "heterosexuals" seek that rare true and lasting fairytale love experience, I believe "homosexuals" seek the same experience. Therefore, it appears the purpose of love, in the minds of pro-homosexuals, is contentment, fulfillment, and happiness, though this purpose is not grounded in God or focused on God at all.

**Comparing and Contrasting**
Some people believe love is the most powerful force in existence. I am inclined to agree with them. Love has the power to change people's hearts and minds, and reorder their entire lives. Love has the power to save people from darkness. Love has the power to penetrate to the core of someone's existence and renew his or her being. This is an impossible task for a mere feeling. This is only possible because God is love. Love is not an idea or a concept; it is something that actually exists. As a result it cannot have conflicting definitions. God's definition of love, which has nothing to do with sex, is entirely contrary to the pro-homosexual concept of love, which is grounded in sex and often defined by sex. The latter is not love at all; it is lust. Lust is obviously sinful, as it violates several of God's commandments, and yet lust is the key foundational element in the "homosexual" lifestyle. Secondly, the Bible says, "Love does no harm to its neighbor" (Romans

13:10), but we've already established homosexuality harms everyone involved. Homosexuality, therefore, cannot be accurately based off of love. An individual can use the term "love" to justify the gratifying of their sexual appetites all they want, but that doesn't mean that it is true. Even "heterosexual" men and women use the word "love" to get sex. In the end, we must remember humans aren't love, God is, and therefore God's definition of love supersedes ours. The attempt to tie love to sex or redefine love in any way is sinful.

# Marriage

The institution of marriage reaches back in history to the first couple that walked the earth, and has existed all over the world in every culture from that day to this. Though the meaning, purpose, and method of marriage vary greatly, it remains the foundational institution in society.

**ACCORDING TO GOD**

*Definition of Marriage*
Marriage is a sacred and holy covenant between a man and a woman that is exclusive and permanent. To fully grasp this definition, we have to also define the word *covenant* because its connotation and significance has been largely lost on us today. A covenant is a solemn and binding promise of great significance. Covenants are sacred in nature, and they are intended to be permanent—never broken by either party. This is foreign to us because we break our word all the time. We say we're going to do things we never do; we make excuses, we forget, and we constantly go back on our promises. This in no way diminishes the significance or sacred nature of covenants. God established many covenants throughout the Bible and He

never broke one of them, which is remarkable because He is an eternal being. God can keep multiple promises for all time, and some of us can't even keep our own promises for a week. All of God's covenants have this in common: they were established out of love and selflessness, they were established for the betterment and protection of a person or group of people, and they were a sign of God's permanent dedication and commitment to that person or group of people.

Here's the key: in establishing covenants God set a specific pattern, a template to be followed, that is grounded in himself. Love and unity are the two key components within each covenant; without love and unity the covenants would not exist. There are three overarching covenants, each one a consistent, complementary, representation of the other two:

1. The covenant established between God and His people—Israel
2. The covenant established between Christ and His church
3. The covenant established between man and his wife.

Consider how God himself describes His covenant with Israel: "For your Maker is your husband—the Lord Almighty is his name" (Isaiah 54:7). Consider how the covenant between Christ and the church is always described in the Bible. "I promised you to one husband, to Christ, so that I might present you as a pure virgin to him" (2 Corinthians 11:2). Jesus is repeatedly described as the bridegroom and the church as his bride. Now consider how the covenant between a man and his wife is related to and perfectly consistent with the previous two:

> Husbands, love your wives just as Christ loved the church and gave himself up for her to make her holy, cleansing her by the

washing with water through the word, and
to present her to himself as a radiant church,
without stain or wrinkle or any other blemish,
but holy and blameless. In the same way, hus-
bands ought to love their wives as their own
bodies. He who loves his wife loves himself.
After all, no one ever hated his own body, but
he feeds and cares for it, just as Christ does
the church—for we are members of his body.
For this reason a man will leave his father and
mother and be united to his wife, and the two
will become one flesh (Ephesians 5:25–31).

Is it not fascinating that here the Apostle Paul quotes the
Scripture in Genesis reaffirming God's definition of marriage, which is exactly what Jesus did when He reaffirmed
God's definition of marriage? Is it not fascinating the covenant between man and wife was the first of the three that was
established, and the other two were designed using it as a
template? This is the profound significance that the covenant
of marriage has to God. Again because God created marriage,
marriage is inherently good, and marriage has a divine purpose that is also good.

*Purpose of Marriage*
The purpose of marriage is to glorify God, to establish a pure
and loving relationship between one man and one woman,
to set the most solid foundation of a family, and to produce
Godly offspring. In addition to the love and unity that allow
marriage to exist and function properly, there is also an undeniable and utterly sacred purity that must be indefinitely maintained. This was emphasized in the aforementioned Scripture
in 2 Corinthians when the church is compared to a pure virgin
to be presented to Christ—her husband. The Bible's emphasis
on purity and virginity in the Bible is key. Hebrews 13:4 says

quite succinctly, "Marriage should be honored by all, and the marriage bed kept pure, for God will judge the adulterer and all the sexually immoral." The covenant must be protected, valued, and must not be broken or defiled by premarital or extramarital sexual encounters of any kind. It must remain pure from its inception on.

## ACCORDING TO PRO-HOMOSEXUALS

*Definition of Marriage*
Defining marriage is more complex for pro-homosexuals. They do not view marriage as a singular institution but a pluralistic institution. Therefore, they divide marriage into primarily two categories, namely "traditional marriage" (marriage between one man and one woman) and "gay marriage." Pro-homosexuals do not deny the legitimacy of "traditional marriage"; however, many of them maintain a negative view of it and claim "traditional marriage" intentionally discriminates against the "LGBT" community. This is what drove the initiative to establish and normalize "gay marriage" and ensure "traditional marriage" is not superior to it in any way. "Gay marriage" is simply defined as the "marriage" between two individuals of the same sex and is often rationalized with the promise that it will have absolutely no effect on the existing institution of marriage. Notice, though, the word *marriage* is included in both the term "gay marriage" and its definition. The word *marriage* obviously has its own definition, and so defining "gay marriage" this way does indeed attempt to redefine marriage itself. Regardless if this is acknowledged or not, pro-homosexuals see the normalization of "gay marriage" as a positive thing, so they are overjoyed now that it has been forced on America despite the overwhelming majority that voted to recognize biblical marriage.

Many pro-homosexuals had passionately joined the fight for "marriage equality," which sought to grant "homosexual" unions the same legal recognition and benefits afforded to "traditional marriages." Achieving this immediately resulted in other issues they were warned about for years now: participants in plural unions such as throuples and quartets have already begun to argue "traditional marriage" and "gay marriage" intentionally discriminate against them and shouldn't be superior to their "marriages" in any way. This is precisely why a larger campaign has been launched under the banner of "gay rights" to define marriage in an even broader sense such as: an inclusive legally recognized union between two or more individuals of any sex. Under this broad definition of marriage, anyone and everyone can get married. However, at that point, marriage has been so radically redefined that one must question if it is necessary at all anymore.

*Purpose of Marriage*
Some pro-homosexuals believe the purpose of marriage is to allow any two people who are in love to solidify their relationship and be equally recognized as any married "heterosexual" couple in society. The picture painted here suggests "traditional marriage" and "gay marriage" are different but should be considered equal. I'm sure you have heard the argument as often as I have: "How does letting homosexuals get married have any effect on you?" or "You're able to have traditional marriage, so we should be able to have 'gay marriage.'" It is important to note that marriage, while undoubtedly the goal of many "homosexuals," is not the goal for all of them. Even with that option now available nationwide, there are many "homosexuals" who have no intentions of ever getting married, and yet they still find purpose for "gay marriage": instead of marriage *being* a destination, it is simply a tool to *reach* a destination. Achieving "marriage equality" was not the end of the fight; the fight continues beyond that to redefining society and legitimizing homosexuality. This leads us to the true objective, the secret agenda hidden behind

the fight for "gay rights" and "marriage equality," which is not to simply redefine marriage but to eliminate marriage altogether. Most pro-homosexuals would never admit this; however, lesbian journalist Masha Gessen unashamedly did. Gessen was one of several participants in a "homosexual" panel discussion for the Sydney Writers Festival, and the question posed by the forum was: why get married when you could be happy? Her response was astonishing. She said, "I agree it's a no-brainer that [homosexuals] should have the right to marry, but I also think equally that it's a no-brainer that the institution of marriage should not exist." This was met with great cheers and applause from the live audience. "That causes my brain some trouble," Gessen continued:

> *...and part of why it causes me trouble is because fighting for gay marriage generally involves lying about what we are going to do with marriage when we get there, because we lie that the institution of marriage is not going to change. And that is a lie. The institution of marriage is going to change, and it should change. And again, I don't think it should exist.*[36]

Though I wholeheartedly disagree with Gessen, I respect her for her candor regarding the lies other "LGBT" activists tell to hide their true intentions regarding marriage. They've made it appear that once all fifty states legally recognize "gay marriage," and "marriage equality" has been achieved, their task will be complete. This is far from true as we are now seeing with more concentrated attacks on ministers, churches, and Christianity as a whole. Their purpose for marriage is merely a means to an end.

## Comparing and Contrasting

Quotations are often added in the term "gay marriage" because it is an oxymoronic term. Marriage has long preceded the concept of "gay marriage," and so the definition and history of marriage must be taken into account. The term "gay marriage," then, is accurately defined as a "homosexual" sacred and holy covenant between a man and a woman that is exclusive and permanent. Or in simpler common vernacular: a "homosexual" "heterosexual" bond. This is totally contradictory and utter nonsense. The fact is, when a man and a woman (which God created) enter into the sacred and permanent covenant (which God created) out of love (which God is and produces) in fulfillment of their unique purposes (which God established) to set the foundation for family (which God created) by having sex (which God designed to be exclusive between a husband and wife), they are honoring God by fulfilling the requirements and purpose for true marriage. Any attempt to redesign or deviate from this pattern is an attempt to remove God from His own design, which is impossible and obviously sinful. Furthermore, marriage is a destination, not a tool to reach a destination. Marriage is born out of love, pure and Godly love, and nothing else. The fruit of marriage is easy to see. Every successful and flourishing society was built on loving and successful marriages because marriage is the key foundational institution in a society. History has taught us that changing or removing that key foundational institution doesn't *enrich* a society, it *crumbles* a society. Peter LaBarbera, president of Americans for Truth about Homosexuality, said, "People suffer and societies crumble when immoral, unhealthy behaviors are not just tolerated, but fostered and even celebrated by the State and corporate/cultural elites."[37]

The reasons for this are both natural and spiritual. It is a fact that "homosexual" couples cannot reproduce. The divine purpose and roles of male and female are impossible to fulfill in "homosexual" relationships. It's impossible for two men, or two women to become one flesh, which is exactly what the key component of marriage is. Consequently "gay marriage" is inherently sinful because it is founded on sinfulness. In addition, any time the holy and sacred covenant of marriage is defiled, redefined, or devalued in any way it is an offense to God, it is a sin, and sin has devastating consequences.

# Sex

How sex works and what it produces is no mystery. Sex is attractive and sex is addictive, which explains the prevalence it has in our culture. The nature of sex has shifted from sacred and private to trivial and overt. "Sex sells," which is why sex, sensuality, and nudity are featured everywhere from commercials, to magazines, to billboards, to movies, to digital images, and that's not including the porn industry. Still, though we have a concept of what sex is and what its purpose is, that does not mean that our concept is accurate or comprehensive.

## ACCORDING TO GOD

*Definition of Sex*
Sex is the physical and spiritual act of consummating a marriage between a husband and wife in the most binding and intimate way. Now the word *consummate* has a few definitions and two are highly relevant here. The first is: to complete the marital bond by having the first sexual marital experience. The second is: to fulfill and bring to a state of perfection. Sex, according to God, is the combination of these two definitions. Sex is a selfless response to absolute love and adoration; it is a priceless gift a husband offers to his wife and a wife offers to her husband simultaneously. This mutual exchange is perfectly pure and brings with it no remnants of previous

sexual encounters. Sex is born out of love within the bonds of marriage, where it matures and remains indefinitely. Love is accentuated and personified in the process, and "the two will become one flesh," as God declared in Genesis, Jesus reaffirmed is the Gospels, and the Apostle Paul reaffirmed in his letters.

Now, can sex take place before and outside of marriage? Obviously it can. In today's society all of the spiritual and Godly attributes of sex are often stripped away until all that remains is the physical act. However, the physical act of sexual intercourse is not the same as the sex God created, because its divine significance is lost entirely when it is done out of order. Sex is defiled and devalued when reduced in any way. Consequently, abusing sex dishonors God, it violates God's will for His creation, and it is therefore sinful. I am well aware this is probably the most disliked aspect of Christianity, because our society is driven by and saturated in sex. Sadly, many Christians who oppose homosexuality based on what the Bible says are sexually immoral themselves. They masturbate, view pornography, and have sex before and outside of marriage as though they are somehow an exception to the rule. I've seen it time and time again: both young Christian men and women are celibate and holy, having vowed to wait until marriage to have sex. Then when they "fall in love" and the opportunity arises, suddenly their attention shifts from honoring God to appeasing themselves with their new boyfriend or girlfriend, they forsake their vow and give their purity away as though it wasn't priceless. Then the process continues indefinitely for every new relationship they enter, as if that pattern is somehow not sexually immoral. Even so, it remains true that God created sex and set specific parameters for it. In following God's design for sex, goodness results and the marital union is blessed. Sexual morality is achieved when all sexual passion flows out of selfless love, and all sexual activity is exclusive to the bonds of marriage:

one hundred percent of the wife's passion and energy is dedicated to her husband, and one hundred percent of the husband's passion and energy is dedicated to his wife. It is only when these conditions are met that sex is pure. By contrast, all other variations and configurations of sexual encounters are impure and sinful.

*Purpose of Sex*

Just as marriage is born of love, sex is born of love in marriage. The purpose of sex is most simply: unity and fruitfulness. Unity results in the selfless expression of the unique love between a husband and wife; the mutual pleasure experienced physically, mentally, emotionally, and spiritually, and in the simultaneous glorification of God through sexual morality, which is most important. Fruitfulness results in not only the strengthening of the marital bond that only sex produces, but also more literally in the producing of offspring. The purpose of sex according to God's design is the only one that reaches *beyond* the two individuals having sex; it points to God, it fulfills the divine purpose for which male and female were created, and it produces children, creating another sacred institution called *family*.

## ACCORDING TO PRO-HOMOSEXUALS

*Definition of Sex*

It is an undeniable fact that the female body and the male body were designed to be sexually compatible. A pair of females and a pair of males are biologically sexually incompatible. This results in all sorts of erotic alternatives to simulate natural sexual relations between a male and a female, and yet pro-homosexuals still call it sex. Based on this, the pro-homosexual definition of sex is: any variety of erotic behaviors between two or more people.

*Purpose of Sex*

"Homosexuals" do not have sex to consummate a marriage because that is impossible. "Homosexuals" do not have sex to produce children because that is also impossible. "Homosexuals" do not have sex to fulfill their divine purpose or glorify God because that is also impossible. The only purposes that remain are pleasure—which is the foremost purpose of homosexuality—and to physically express one's romantic feelings for an individual of the same gender. The reason for this is homosexuality is lust driven, not God driven. God is the source of purpose, and removing God from sex also removes His divine purpose for sex. Beyond that, it attempts to redefine every aspect of God's design in order to satisfy one's sexual desires uninhibited by anything or anyone. The purpose of "homosexual" sex never goes beyond the individuals engaging in the erotic acts. This selfish purpose of pursing pleasure fails to glorify God in any way and therefore falls into the category of sexual immorality. This, and the fact that it is unnatural, abnormal, and a violation of God's design, is precisely why "homosexual" "sex" is entirely sinful.

**Comparing and Contrasting**

Consider this analogy to underscore what we've learned thus far: the key was created with a specific purpose, as was the lock. The key fits perfectly into its counterpart, and the two together fulfill the purpose for which they were created, namely to secure something of value. Now, can you put two keys together? Sure, but neither key will fulfill the purpose for which it was created by doing so. Can you put two locks together? Of course, but neither lock will fulfill the purpose for which it was created by doing so. Only when the key works with its complementary counterpart—the lock—does the key fulfill its purpose, the lock fulfills its purpose, and the greater purpose of securing something valuable is fulfilled. The greater purpose is more valuable than either the key or the lock themselves, but together in the fulfillment of their purpose there is tremendous value. By comparing the definitions and purposes of sex according to God and sex according to pro-homosexuals, it becomes quite clear the latter is sinful from its inception. Homosexuality violates God's commands in multiple ways: it violates the goodness and purpose of sex, it cannot possibly take place within the bonds of marriage, it is entirely selfish in nature because it fails to serve any purpose beyond the individuals having "sex," it is driven by lust, the primary objective is experiencing pleasure not obedience to God, and it results in a plethora of negative, spiritual, and physical consequences, including death. God's design and purpose for sex are perfect, and everything outside of God's design and purpose for sex is imperfect, dangerous, and sinful.

# Family

Family means different things to different people. As we've already discovered, our individual perceptions are not necessarily accurate or comprehensive, nor do they apply to everyone. Thus, we must also take an objective look at family to discern its true definition and purpose.

## ACCORDING TO GOD

*Definition of Family*
Family is a group of relatives consisting of a man, his wife, and their offspring. Two individuals who love God above all else, who love each other as they love themselves, and are totally committed to each other for life set the best foundation for parenthood. This is not only a spiritual principle; it is a natural principle as well. The beautiful thing about God's design for mankind is when we are obedient and remain in

God's will, everyone benefits and experiences the best results. When love comes first, then marriage, then sex, the proper foundation for a family is already established when children follow. This, of course, was done by design. In the end the bond between all members of the family is unique and strong, as are every member's personal relationship with God.

*Purpose of Family*
The purpose of family is to glorify God, to grow in love and support, to raise Godly offspring, and to understand God even better. Family is about children. Marriage obviously remains a priority, but the mutual priority of both husband and wife becomes the nurturing, developing, teaching, protecting, and loving their offspring. As God created man in His image, children are created in the likeness of their parents and share their same genetics, talents, and appearance. Since God is our heavenly Father, the experience of having children produces feelings and emotions that parents never knew they could have, which broadens their understanding and appreciation of God.

I heard a husband confess after he and his wife experienced childbirth for the first time, he suddenly realized he loved his wife more than ever before—something he never knew was possible. In addition, his love for his child was indescribable. Together the bond between himself and his wife and the bond between parents and child were stronger than he could have imagined was possible. This, of course, was also God's design. The transition from husband, to husband and father, and from wife, to wife and mother is an amazing experience that paints an even clearer picture of *how* God loves us and how *much* God loves us as our heavenly Father.

## ACCORDING TO PRO-HOMOSEXUALS

*Definition of Family*
Family is a group comprised of two or more parental figures and at least one child. Gone is the traditional idea of a mother and father with children in a home. "Modern families" now include two fathers or two mothers who raise children. This poses an obvious problem for "homosexual" couples because as we've already pointed out, it is impossible for "homosexual" couples to naturally produce children. To remedy this there are several alternatives "homosexual" couples are forced to rely on to create families. Some simply adopt children; others use surrogates to compensate for the missing female, or sperm donors to compensate for the missing male in order to create life. There are actually medical facilities that allow "homosexual" couples to request what sex they would like their child to be beforehand. "Homosexual" males will provide sperm to a willing surrogate, who will give birth and then sacrifice her role as a mother and give the child to the "homosexual" couple. "Lesbians" have even devised a workaround, where one woman is artificially inseminated with the sperm of her partner's brother in order to produce a child who carries the DNA of both females. When this happens, in addition to having two moms as parents, the child will also have an "uncle" who is literally their father. Masha Gessen also touched on this issue at the previously referenced "homosexual" panel. She said:

> *I have three kids who have five parents, more or less, and I don't see why they shouldn't have five parents legally. I don't see why we should choose two of those parents and make them into a sanctioned couple . . . I got married in Massachusetts to my partner who is Russian, my ex-partner, and by that time we*

*had two kids, one of whom was adopted and one of whom I gave birth to. We broke up a couple years after that, and a couple years after that I met my new partner, and she [had] just had a baby, and that baby's biological father is my brother, and my daughter's biological father is a man who lives in Russia, and my adopted son also considers him his father. So the five parents break down into two groups of three who have two different citizenships. And really, I would like to live in a legal system that is capable of reflecting that reality, and I don't think that's compatible with the institution of marriage.*

As you can see, instead of the traditional family structure this idea of family includes any number of individuals, many who aren't related by blood, who serve multiple customized roles, which is incredibly confusing, unstable, and often dysfunctional as a result.

*Purpose of Family*
Because a "homosexual" does not enter into the divinely created role of husband or wife in marriage, that does not necessarily negate their innate desire to be a parent. Also, it is often the desire for "homosexual" couples to further mirror the institutions of "heterosexuals." So in addition to inventing "gay marriage" to emulate "traditional marriage," they've also invented "modern families" to emulate "traditional families" in an effort to prove "homosexual" couples are equally suitable for raising children. The extra "benefit" to this is it ensures "homosexuals" are able to expose their children to their ideology and way of life in order to raise them as "homosexuals" or at the least advocates. Another underlying purpose of family is the need to feel loved. Many

"homosexuals" have admittedly identified the source of their sexual confusion as a lack of love in their own lives from their parents, siblings, or other family members. This has resulted in a void that many "homosexuals" have tried and failed to fill in many ways. The love of a child is one of the ways some seek to fill that void, and in the process some "homosexuals" vow to raise their children in such a way that they never experience the same problematic upbringing.

**Comparing and Contrasting:**
The primary divine focus of family is children. The primary pro-homosexual focus of family is same-sex parents. The goal of the latter is not to provide the best possible conditions for a child to grow, develop, and be trained in a moral and godly home to be moral and godly individuals. By removing God and His design for family the pro-homosexual goal for family is reduced to a selfish desire. The fact is there are certain lessons that no one can teach better than a mother, certain values that no one can instill better than a mother, and certain precepts and examples that only a mother can set. Therefore, to remove the mother from a child is immediately creating a void that may never be filled outside of Christ. There is no relationship like the one between mother and son and the one between mother and daughter. It simply cannot be mimicked or replaced by a second "father." Likewise, there are certain lessons that no one can teach better than a father, certain values that no one can instill better than a father, and certain precepts and examples that only a father can set. There is simply no relationship like the one between father and son and the one between father and daughter. It simply cannot be mimicked or replaced by a second "mother." We've seen the results of removing the father from a child time and time again, and the void that it creates in young men and women is harrowing. Whether it's a celebrity opening up about their fatherless upbringing or a young man in jail detailing his

childhood without knowing who his father is, the hurt and anger expressed in these stories are unlike any other. Think about how many people grow up without their mother or father and spend years, sometimes decades, searching for them, hoping to fill that void. I've seen this firsthand and it is not a pleasant sight. The blend of pain, emptiness, and sense of loneliness that results from growing up and living apart from one's biological parent is devastating. God never intended for any of us to experience such misery, so we certainly shouldn't be creating and supporting situations that foster that sort of misery. Don't take my word for it. Consider the sobering words of a young lady who was raised by "lesbians" named Katy Faust:

> *Talk to any child with gay parents, especially those old enough to reflect on their experiences. If you ask a child raised by a lesbian couple if they love their two moms, you'll probably get a resounding "yes!" Ask about their father, and you are in for either painful silence, a confession of gut wrenching longing, or the recognition that they have a father that they wish they could see more often. The one thing that you will not hear is indifference. What is your experience with children who have divorced parents, or are the offspring of third-party reproduction, or the victims of abandonment? Do they not care about their missing parent? Do those children claim to have never had a sleepless night wondering why their parents left, what they look like, or if they love their child? Of course not. We are made to know, and be known by, both of our parents. When one is absent, that absence leaves a lifelong gaping*

*wound. The opposition will clamor on about studies where the researchers concluded that children in same-sex households allegedly fared "even better!" than those from intact biological homes. Leave aside the methodological problems with such studies and just think for a moment. If it is undisputed social science that children suffer greatly when they are abandoned by their biological parents, when their parents divorce, when one parent dies, or when they are donor-conceived, then how can it be possible that they are miraculously turning out "even better!" when raised in same-sex-headed households? Every child raised by "two moms" or "two dads" came to that household via one of those four traumatic methods. Does being raised under the rainbow miraculously wipe away all the negative effects and pain surrounding the loss and daily deprivation of one or both parents? The more likely explanation is that researchers are feeling the same pressure as the rest of us feel to prove that they love their gay friends.*[38]

God's design for family is not only clear; it is proven successful. Numerous studies have been conducted in various countries around the world, and the results are conclusive: the children in "homosexual" households do not fare equal to or better than children in a biological heterosexual household; they consistently fare worse. While children in intact families raised by a mother and father who are married excel and develop healthily and strong mentally, physically, and emotionally, they also perform better in school and society. In comparison, children of "homosexual" couples do not develop as well, they suffer mentally, emotionally, and physically, they do not excel as much, nor do their performances in school and society exceed the children in traditional families. Mexican sociologist Fernando Pliego examined an incredible amount of data from studies gathered from thirteen democratic countries.

> Professor Pliego concluded that the natural family was far superior to other forms. He found that 89.4 percent of the studies concluded that intact families produced a higher level of well-being than other family types. . . . That is to say, the natural family has been clearly demonstrated by social science to be superior to all other forms.[39]

Pain, emptiness, and dysfunction are the results of attempting to redesign God's plans for mankind, love, sex, marriage, and family. Before, there was an understandable silence from those individuals who had negative experiences growing up in a same-sex household, but we are now starting to hear from more and more adults like Katy who are boldly sharing their unpleasant experiences in an effort to discourage "gay marriage" and same-sex parenting.

### Heather Barwick:

*Same-sex marriage and parenting withholds either a mother or father from a child while telling him or her that it doesn't matter. That it's all the same. But it's not. A lot of us, a lot of your kids, are hurting. My father's absence created a huge hole in me, and I ached every day for a dad. I loved my mom's partner, but another mom could never have replaced the father I lost.[40]*

## B. N. Klein:

*I grew up with a parent and her partner[s] in an atmosphere in which gay ideology was used as a tool of repression, retribution and abuse. I have seen that children in gay households often become props to be publicly displayed to prove that gay families are just like heterosexual ones.*[41]

## Robert Oscar Lopez:

*I had an inexplicable compulsion to have sex with older males. [I] wanted to have sex with older men who were my father's age, though at the time I could scarcely understand what I was doing. . . . My re-establishment of ties to my father in 1998 led to a transition in my life, from being lost and sexually confused to being stable and romantically fulfilled.*[40]

## Dawn Stefanowicz:

*I wasn't surrounded by average heterosexual couples. Dad's partners slept and ate in our home, and they took me along to meeting places in the "LGBT" communities. I was exposed to overt sexual activities like sodomy, nudity, pornography, group sex, sadomasochism and the ilk. There was no guarantee that any of my Dad's partners would be around for long, and yet I often had to obey them. My rights and innocence were violated.*[40]

Accounts such as these are both tragic and powerful as they come directly from the source – the individuals who have experienced it firsthand. To my great astonishment, there are people who are so pro-homosexual and such advocates for "gay marriage" and same-sex parenting, that they pretend these personal testimonies are inconsequential. What's interesting to note is every single person I know who argues for same-sex parenting was not raised by same-sex parents. Yet they believe their opinions somehow supersede the personal accounts of those who were raised by same-sex parents. In one discussion, after a young lady I know professed her support for same-sex parenting, I informed her of the harm these children suffer citing specific examples like the ones I've provided here. Her response? "There's two sides to every story." Can you believe that? A young lady, who enjoyed the fruits of being raised by both of her biological parents, insinuated that the children who suffered from same-sex parenting are mistaken or even lying! It's quite astonishing how far some people will go to ignore any reality that conflicts with their preconceived notions.

People can put on smiles and present these "modern families" as progressive and loving, but the fact is that they are damaging because they are flawed. They are built upon sin and cannot flourish as a result. This is simply unacceptable for our children. Children are an invaluable priority in life. They rely on us to provide them with God's best to give them the best chance of succeeding in life. We do them a tremendous disservice when we attempt to rework God's design and force them to accept anything less than the best. We do them a tremendous disservice by raising them in conditions that cause them harm. In "homosexual" couples the child is robbed of a mother or a father one hundred percent of the time. Group raising fails to match or exceed a mother and a father raising their child together. These customized families not only fail to perform the best on a natural level, they fail on a spiritual level because they are built outside of God's good and perfect will. It is only when a child is raised by both a mother and father that they can be truly complete and develop in the proper setting with the proper love the way

God intended for them to. Goodness, success, and blessings are the result of following God's perfect design for family.

# Summary

So what have we learned here? Because God is perfect and the highest form of good, He cannot make mistakes, and He is inevitably the standard by which all things are judged. Anything that is like God is good; anything that is unlike God is evil. Whenever one attempts to change, redefine, or reject God's will, they are committing a sin. Mankind was created to know good, to do good, and to be good. Remember God's desire was for mankind to never even know what evil was. In the beginning Adam and Eve were blessed and protected and wanted for absolutely nothing. Their first mistake was in questioning God. They fell prey to Satan's deception and adopted his precedent of questioning God's goodness by asking: "Did God really say…?" This resulted in disobedience (which is evil in itself), and the consequences were catastrophic. We do the same thing today. We read God's commandments and still ask, "Did God really say…?" We resist God's goodness, question God's goodness, and disobey God in order to satisfy ourselves as though our own desires and our knowledge are somehow superior to God's. This sinful behavior simply cannot be tolerated in a creation that was never intended to know evil let alone indulge in it. As it relates to homosexuality, in every creation we've discussed (mankind, love, marriage, sex, and family) there is a direct conflict between God's purpose for His creation, and the pro-homosexual concept of these creations. Again, anything outside of God's good and perfect will is evil. Evil is another word for sin or sinfulness. In rejecting God there is sin, in disobeying God there is sin, in idolatry (which is loving anything or anyone more than God) there is sin, in sexual immorality (the basis of the entire "homosexual" lifestyle) there is sin. Considering this, it becomes abundantly clear why homosexuality violates God's Moral Law and is therefore considered sinful.

So despite the adamant assertion of activists like Matthew Vines that "gay Christians" exist (meaning practicing "homosexuals" who profess Christianity), they are mistaken because there is no such thing as a "sinner Christian." There are no exceptions to God's designs. So the question, "what about loving committed Christian 'gay marriages'?" is a loaded question because it ignores that fact that homosexuality is inherently sinful, and it presupposes that in the presence of love and commitment, there is an absence of sin. It also suggests God's design for human sexuality and marriage is imperfect and can include same-sex unions. This is all clearly false and is merely an attempt to rationalize homosexuality by manipulating facts and Scripture. The results remain the same: God does not approve of homosexuality in any fashion, and therefore God does not approve of "homosexual" unions of any fashion, regardless if there is love and commitment or not.

Now imagine for a moment what would happen if everyone in the world agreed with God regarding His definitions and divine purposes for mankind, love, marriage, sex, and family. What would that world look like? STDs wouldn't exist, nor would divorce, adultery, broken families, children born out of wedlock, abortions, lust, rape, masturbation, pedophilia, incest, bestiality, pornography, depression, or violence. There would be no erotic behavior between members of the same sex. There would be no such thing as mental, physical, or sexual abuse. There would be no physical damage suffered from violating God's design for the human body. There would be no sexual immorality of any kind. In this world God's will would be done in the lives of everyone.

There would be purity in all relationships, respect and honor for all of God's creations and the parameters He's set for each of His creations. The endless pursuit of sinful pleasure would be replaced with the endless pursuit of God. I believe if we want to shift our culture toward something progressive and modern and loving, *this* is what we should be fighting for. Not sinful lifestyles that reject and offend God and damage all involved in order to indulge in boundless sexual exploits.

# 7

## What Is the True Christian Position on Homosexuality?

The current Christian response to homosexuality is all over the place. If you ask a hundred Christians to affirm the true Christian position on homosexuality, instead of getting the same answer a hundred times, you would likely get a hundred different answers. How can this be if we are all members of the body of Christ who serve the same God, mirror the same Savior, read the same Bible, and are led by the same Holy Spirit? Something is obviously amiss.

This lack of consensus among Christians is one of the primary reasons there is so much confusion surrounding homosexuality. Tragically, when we observe Christian leadership (the group that exists to provide spiritual clarity and direction) we find just as much dissension! Today's most prominent evangelists and megachurch pastors influence untold millions with their contradictory messages. On one end of the spectrum are individuals such as evangelist Franklin Graham. Historically Graham has consistently and fearlessly taught the biblical truth that homosexuality is sinful, and he continues to do so now despite our increasingly pro-homosexual culture. On the opposite end of the spectrum are false teachers such as Jim Swilley, the twice married father of four, who not only *endorses* homosexuality, he *practices* homosexuality. Swilley, a megachurch pastor, shocked his congregation when he announced he is "gay." Later he divorced his wife of twenty-one years. He is currently "married" to another man and he believes (and teaches) that God embraces homosexuality. Another false teacher at this end of the spectrum is Eddie Long. Long was a megachurch pastor who was renowned for vigorously opposing homosexuality. He was forced to step down after getting caught in a dreadful scandal where he preyed on teenage boys (several from his own congregation) using money and gifts to lure them into sexual relationships. Somewhere in the middle of the spectrum are the many evangelists and pastors who remain utterly silent on homosexuality to avoid any controversy. To make matters worse, there are those who send mixed and misleading messages that only add to the confusion. For example, Bishop T.D. Jakes recently sparked a firestorm of controversy after an interview where he described his thoughts on homosexuality as "evolved and evolving." The backlash from Christians and conservatives was so severe that Jakes felt obligated to clarify his remarks not once, but twice in an effort to convince everyone that he does not endorse homosexuality. Less publicized were Jakes' misleading remarks from the same interview concerning "homosexuals" and the church:

> *Every church has a different opinion on the*
> *issue and every gay person is different. LGBTs*
> *of different types and sorts have to find a place*
> *of worship that reflects what your views are*
> *and what you believe like anyone else. And*
> *the church should have the right to have its*

> *own convictions and values. If you don't like*
> *those convictions and values, you totally dis-*
> *agree with it, don't try to change my house;*
> *move into your own, and establish that sort*
> *of thing, and find somebody who gets what*
> *you get about faith, and, trust me, I've talked*
> *to enough LGBT and they're not all the same.*

I am still astonished by this garbled statement. Not only is it incoherent, Jakes did not encourage "LGBT" individuals to seek a church that loves them enough to tell them the *truth* based on *God's word*. Instead he encouraged them to seek a church that teaches what they already believe about homosexuality! How absurd is that? Sadly, because Jakes is such a prominent Christian figure, his recommendation was undoubtedly taken as gospel. There's no telling how many people sought out churches that embrace homosexuality and felt justified in doing so because of Jakes' erroneous message.

This is just a glimpse of the problem. Should we be surprised by confused flocks when we see they are led by confused shepherds? Not at all. Christian leaders do the church and the world a great disservice when they do not stand together united on the foundation of Scriptural truth, and guide people toward God and away from sin. Sure, churches *can* establish their own convictions and values, but that doesn't mean they align with God's word. Churches are *obligated* to establish convictions and values that align with God's word; otherwise they are not true churches. We must not be dissuaded by politically correct rhetoric and lose sight of the truth: there is only one true Christian position on homosexuality; all the other "Christian positions" are false. Professing Christians fall into four major categories: the hateful opponents, the neutrals, the loving proponents, and the loving opponents. Examining these categories will reveal the true Christian position on homosexuality.

# Hateful Opponents of Homosexuality

Those who fall into this category fail to separate the sinfulness of homosexuality from the people engaging in homosexuality. They take great offense to both homosexuality *and* "homosexuals" and make harsh statements like, "All gays are going to hell!" and "God hates gays!" They often use hateful, derogatory terms in place of "gay," or "homosexual." What's worse is these people actually believe they are doing the right thing. They are actually convinced God wants them to condemn all "homosexuals" and somehow using an entirely negative approach will have some kind of positive effect. They couldn't be more mistaken, and their position is actually anti-Christian. I have never in my life heard of a practicing "homosexual" being screamed at, condemned, and called all sorts of derogatory names by a "Christian" who then replied, "You're right. I renounce my life of homosexuality, and I will now become a Christian like you." On the contrary, it seems the primary goal of the hateful opposer is to hurt "homosexuals" instead of helping them. They focus entirely on pointing the finger at "homosexuals" instead of pointing the finger at the solution to homosexuality. As such, the hateful opposers are terribly misguided, misinformed, and cause considerable damage not only to the "homosexuals" who are seeking help, but to the true body of Christ that deplores such hateful, anti-Christian tactics.

# The Neutral Position on Homosexuality

Those who choose a neutral position straddle the fence as a means of avoidance. Their primary objective is not to help "homosexuals" but to avoid arguments, controversy, uncomfortable situations, and the possibility of offending people.

They believe if they take a firm position either way, they won't be able to avoid these things. What is most ironic is the majority of neutrals I know, who wish to avoid arguments about homosexuality, actually go around starting arguments with anyone who is not neutral on the subject! In their minds it's okay to remain silent and avoid an important issue like homosexuality to avoid arguments, but it's quite alright to chastise those who do speak out against homosexuality even if it's done in an entirely respectful way. This is a hypocritical position. Those who aren't quick to argue while trying to avoid arguing often rely on the "I don't know" position like Pastor Chris. Those who are confused also fall into this category. They are simply too confused by the issue to make an intelligible decision either way. I took part in one online discussion about homosexuality where one Christian actually said, "I'm for gay marriage, even though I'm against homosexuality." How confusing and misguided is that? I've heard other Christians say, "What they do in the privacy of their own homes is their business." This is a neutral statement that helps no one and ignores the fact that deplorable sinful behavior frequently goes on in the privacy of people's homes. Remember the previously mentioned "homosexual" couple who bought that baby boy? The horrible abuse they subjected that child to was done in the privacy of their own home. We also cannot forget the long list of horrible, often permanent, effects people suffer from engaging in homosexuality. I guarantee if we were able to glimpse the future and saw our loved ones contract a deadly disease or get diagnosed with cancer or incontinence from privately indulging in homosexuality, we would do everything we could to save them before that became a reality. Even more importantly, if we caught a glimpse of Judgment Day and saw that our loved ones' private actions result in their eternal destruction, we would not rest until we saved them from themselves. It would be immoral to just remain silent and let our loved ones destroy themselves and others.

Secondly, remember the primary objective of the "gay rights" campaign is not to keep homosexuality private, but to publicize and normalize it. This is what "gay pride" and "out and proud" and the pushing of acceptance and tolerance are all about. Gay pride parades aren't private, nor are the "homosexuals" who have been testing the boundaries by going into public establishments and making out in front of everyone to see if someone "discriminates" against them by asking them to stop. If such "discrimination" takes place, they respond by punishing those individuals and establishments with lawsuits, boycotts, threats, and smear campaigns.

Lastly, private immorality is still immorality. Christians are called to be moral and to help save the immoral, so as Christians our focus can't be on avoiding difficult conversations. We can't afford to take the easy road and remain silent or continue saying, "I don't know" to remain neutral, particularly when Jesus himself never took neutral positions when it came to sinfulness. In fact, Jesus said, "I know your deeds, that you are neither cold nor hot. I wish you were either one or the other! So, because you are lukewarm—neither hot nor cold—I am about to spit you out of my mouth" (Revelation 3:15-16). So for any Christian to take a neutral position on homosexuality is obviously to take an incorrect and dangerous position.

## Loving Proponents of Homosexuality

Those in this category, although contrary to the hateful opponents of homosexuality, often cause just as much damage, if not more. Loving proponents of homosexuality are also deceived but in an entirely different way. Most often their position is based on entirely fallacious reasoning that goes like this:

1. To disapprove of homosexuality is hateful.
2. I'm not a hateful person.
3. Therefore I approve of homosexuality.

This rationality is totally illogical because it begins with a false premise. To disapprove of homosexuality is not hateful if done with love and respect. Therefore the conclusion they reach is also false. Nevertheless, they fail to recognize this and passionately defend homosexuality in an effort to promote love over "hatred." Their goal is not to help save the souls of practicing "homosexuals." Their goal is to prevent "homosexuals" from being discriminated against. Loving proponents view "homosexuals" as victims, and they dedicate themselves to standing in the gap to defend them against "bullies." This includes those who challenge homosexuality, but aren't hateful or discriminatory in any way. Loving proponents believe in love to the degree that it not only extends to the individual, but to the sinfulness of that individual. This is obviously dangerous and totally anti-Christian. If you've ever witnessed the journey of an alcoholic, a drug addict, a chain smoker, or a morbidly obese person, you are aware they weren't saved from themselves by ignoring and defending their addictions. On the contrary, the people who loved them the most loved them enough to say, "You have a problem and if you don't change, you will suffer through life and eventually die from this. I don't want you to die so I am going to help you in any way I can." Loving proponents don't say this to "homosexuals." They enable, and excuse, and rationalize sinfulness for the sake of sparing feelings. They do not listen to God's instruction on how we are to treat our neighbors; they do not follow Jesus' command for us to preach the Good News to the entire world, or to rebuke our brother if he sins. The irony is if they were the sinner, and they knew a friend or family member had the solution to save them from eternal damnation but never offered it to them, they would be furious. Saving lives and souls is what it means to love others as we love ourselves.

If you loved yourself enough to secure your own salvation, shouldn't you love your neighbors enough to see their salvation is secured as well? Instead of doing what God commanded them to do, loving proponents *imagine* what God would want them to do. They question the validity of God's Word, they lean to their own understanding, and they ignore the Bible. They accept and defend practicing "homosexuals" with rationalizations like, "Who am I to judge? Only God can judge them." First of all, if you are a Christian and the individual struggling with homosexuality is also a Christian, then you are obligated to judge them. Again, in judging them it isn't the negative, hypocritical, self-righteous action that most people limit judging to. It's merely recognizing your brother or sister is embracing sinfulness, and you're committed to doing whatever is necessary to save them from that sinfulness. That is what Christ did, and that is what Christians are supposed to do for each other. Secondly, to ignore someone's sinful practice instead of trying to save him or her from that sinful practice and saying, "Only God can judge them," is not loving. I wonder how these people would feel on the Day of Judgment when they stand before God's throne and He asks them, "Why did you not believe my word? Why did you ignore the sinfulness of your brothers and sisters instead of helping to save them from it? I put you in their lives to help them, and yet you opted to encourage them in their sinfulness instead." I wonder what they will say then. I wonder what they will say if they happen to witness the judgment of practicing "homosexuals" who never truly accepted God because they embraced sinfulness all their lives. How will these loving proponents respond when they witness the judgment they said only God was fit for? Will they regret seeing these sinners they know and love cast into eternal damnation because no one stood in the gap to rescue them from themselves? Will these loving proponents enter the kingdom of heaven themselves after refusing to follow God's commands? It is the world, those who embrace sin and live in darkness, that defends and promotes homosexuality. How then can Christians do the same thing? How can Christians make a difference if our message is the same as the world's message? We can't afford to be like the world or even think like the world, lest we be led astray like the world. This is the problem with the loving proponents: they don't consider God's will superior to their own will. Consequently, they don't allow themselves to be transformed in Christ or their minds to be renewed. This is why loving proponents, while they mean well, are misguided and have taken the wrong position.

## Loving Opponents of Homosexuality

Loving opponents of homosexuality recognize ultimately this equation has little to do with themselves; it has everything to do with Christ and the individuals who need Christ. We love God above all else, we love our neighbors as ourselves, and consequently we keep in mind that our opinions, thoughts, and understanding are all irrelevant. God's Word is what is relevant, and just as many of us were called out of darkness through the loving persistence of a Christian, we are now focused on pleasing God and calling others out of darkness with the grace and love of Christ. Christ never condoned sinful behavior. Instead, with love and respect, He always helped the lost and told them to leave their life of sin. As Christians our responsibility is to follow Christ's precept and example. We accept the lost with open arms, speak the truth to them in love, and we help them as often and as much as we are able. This is precisely what Christ would still be doing if He were physically here on earth, but since He is still here spiritually within us, the body of Christ continues to reach the lost in His name. This is the proper Christian position regarding homosexuality and every other sinful lifestyle.

# Conclusion

As you can see, there is such inconsistency among professing Christians on the issue of homosexuality that the message Christians present to the world is also inconsistent. Instead of providing healing and clarity, this causes more damage and confusion. Truth is consistent, effective, and necessary. The proper Christian stance on homosexuality, therefore, follows the same pattern by being true, consistent, and effective because it's absolutely necessary. So what is the true Christian position on homosexuality? Should we be shunning and condemning "homosexuals" to hell like the hateful opponents of homosexuality? Should we remain quiet and avoid the issue like those in the neutral category? Should our focus be on loving and defending homosexuality, instead of loving "homosexuals" and defending God's Word like the loving proponents of homosexuality? Or should we be focused entirely on reaching the lost by extending the love of Christ to "homosexuals"? The first category fails in that it rightfully agrees with God that homosexuality is sinful, but it completely removes love and respect from the equation. The second category fails on both counts because they do not stand firm on God's Word by agreeing with it, nor do they practice love by communicating God's Word to those who need it most. The third group fails because they wrongfully disagree with God that homosexuality is sinful but try to express love in spite of that, while not realizing love is empty without God's Word. Therefore, instead of saving the lost through the love of

Christ, they don't save anyone. Yet they believe they're doing right by enabling sinfulness. It is only in the last category that both requirements of agreement with God and expressing Godly love are met. Therefore, the true Christian position on homosexuality is to first agree with God that homosexuality is sinful, and secondly to treat "homosexuals" with love and respect—to be a shining example of a Christian by sharing the truth with love as led by the Holy Spirit.

## The Process

How is this done? Once we agree with God, and we are led by the Holy Spirit to help someone who is caught up in the "homosexual" lifestyle, what do we say? This is a great question and something you definitely want to think about before you find yourself in this situation. The trouble is that most people, though well meaning, resort to spewing out Bible verses and using little catchphrases and imagine this approach will have some sort of life-changing impact. That is rarely the case. I'll give you an example to illustrate why this fails. One of the things I dislike most about talking to aggressive salesmen is how obvious it is they don't care about *me* nearly as much as they care about what they can get *from* me. Their primary mission isn't to help me; it's to make a sale, and the more money they can get from me, the better. Whether or not I'm better off in the end is irrelevant. I'm sure you've experienced this before. This brand of salesman talks fast and throws a lot of information at you at once in an effort to manipulate you. They aim to convince you that they're doing you some great favor, when in fact they're trying to make the biggest sale as fast as possible before moving on to the next person to do it again. While this approach might work in the sales industry, it has no place in sharing the gospel with the lost.

Given this, loading your proverbial machine gun with Bible verses and one-liners and firing away whenever the topic of homosexuality arises can actually do more damage than good. Catchphrases can be especially damaging because the odds are that your "homosexual" loved one has already heard them countless times. "God made Adam and Eve, not Adam and Steve," is one example. It rhymes; it makes a point, but is that what a struggling "homosexual" needs to hear in order to get at the root of the issue? Not quite. "We love the sinner but hate the sin," is another. It's true, that is what we do, but does that solve a sinner's problem? Not at all. Finally, suggesting they "just pray the gay away" is another one that rhymes and people feel it's both cute and effective; I don't believe it's either. None of these catchphrases sound natural; they all run the risk of sounding silly, and homosexuality is not a silly issue or something to be made light of. So I would highly recommend avoiding all such catchphrases.

Oftentimes we want to help so badly that we immediately start talking and sharing our opinions, or start spouting Bible verses. This turns people away instead of drawing them closer to God. Before saying a word, pray and ask God to help you to listen to your "homosexual" loved one, and then give you the words they need to hear to help them. Listening first is a sign of true respect. It shows we understand not all "homosexuals" are alike, not all "homosexuals" have the same struggles, the same history, or are in the same place in life. Therefore, a blanket catchphrase, or merely listing Scriptures is inapplicable and inappropriate here. We need to listen, understand who they are, what they've gone through, how they feel, and where their heart is *first*. Then the Holy Spirit will help us by giving us the words to say in response. That doesn't mean it will be an entire speech. Sometimes it's as simple as, "I heard what you said, and I want to let you know I truly love you. God loves you far more than me and wants nothing more than for you to be free from darkness so you can be with Him. I'm here to help you in any way I can to ensure that happens." Other times it might just take a sincere hug so they can feel the true love of Christ from someone with no hidden agenda.

I came to know an awesome woman who started attending our church and was present the morning I spoke on homosexuality. Afterward, she pulled me aside and confessed she is a "lesbian." She thanked me for my message and told me although she's not out of the lifestyle yet, she's working on it every day. She said, "The only thing I can do is the next right thing."

I totally agreed with her, so I simply thanked her and said, "I hope you know that I love you," and gave her a hug.

She said, "I know. That's the reason that I'm here. I know the difference between real love and fake love, and there is real love at this church."

I was blown away by how much she'd gleaned from a simple logical message spoken in the true love of Christ. This, my brothers and sisters, is how we can save lives, and if we all come together and are unified under one message of truth and love, the body of Christ could have a *phenomenal* impact on a far greater scale. It is my prayer we do exactly that.

# 8

## Why Can Some "Gays" Go "Straight" but Not Others?

**P**erhaps you are a compassionate Christian who desires to help lead your "homosexual" loved ones out of homosexuality but don't know the solution. Perhaps you struggle with homosexuality yourself and can't seem to find the way out. In either case, you've probably asked, why have so many been able to successfully abandon homosexuality while others have tried so hard for so long but failed? I believe, as we've seen thus far, that it is necessary to take a logical, rational approach to properly answer this question.

Any good sports coach will lead their team to victory by not only teaching them how to do what is right but also by teaching them how not to do what is wrong. Both elements are crucial to success. Even if a team wins a game by a blowout but made foolish errors along the way, a good coach won't ignore those foolish errors and focus on the win because those errors could cause them to lose future games. It is the same with life issues such as homosexuality. We must understand the ways in which people fail to overcome homosexuality as well as the ways in which people succeed in overcoming homosexuality so we can fully understand what leads to failure and what leads to success. We will begin with a real-life example of each followed by detailed descriptions of what worked, what didn't work, and why.

# Failure Story

Vicky Beeching is a thirty-five-year-old British Christian rock star who announced she is a "lesbian." In the setup piece of a televised interview, Vicky described how she first experienced SSA at age thirteen and how distressing that was particularly being raised in a Christian family. She sought to cure herself of "lesbianism" by first going to a Catholic priest. She described the encounter in an interview: "When I said that I had feelings for the same sex, he prayed the prayer of absolution for me to be forgiven. And that was it." When that failed, she said it "only increased the sense of shame. I felt there was something really wrong with me, that maybe I was so sinful and awful I couldn't be healed."

Vicky reasoned it was impossible to be both "gay" and Christian, and since she had no interest in renouncing Christianity, her only options were to either die or to be liberated from her "homosexual" feelings. The inner conflict was so distressing, she cried out to God with an ultimatum: "You have to either take my life or take this attraction away because I cannot do both."

God didn't take either her life or her "homosexual" feelings away. Vicky describes the next attempt to solve her problem as an exorcism. While visiting a Christian youth camp, one of the messages was about deliverance, and afterward there was an open invitation for anyone who needed prayer. Vicky accepted and soon there was a group of people laying hands on her, praying loudly, commanding Satan to let her go and the "demon of homosexuality" to release her. When this too failed, Vicky's struggle intensified. Nothing she tried changed anything, and so she turned her focus toward work. Later, although she became a successful Christian musician, she felt increasingly convicted performing Christian songs in Christian venues, all while hiding a sinful secret.

So at the age of thirty-five, having thought about her sexuality "every day," Vicky came to a series of conclusions. She determined her "homosexual" inclinations are from God, she claims she was born "gay," and she claims it is her calling to help other "Christian gay people" to "come out" so they don't have to suffer the turmoil she did.

I watched a heavily slanted news segment[42] in favor of homosexuality that was framed as a debate between Vicky and reverend Scott Lively, whose sister is an "ex-lesbian." This "debate" was essentially a sounding board to promote Vicky and homosexuality while simultaneously painting opponents of homosexuality in a bad light. Unfortunately, Lively was barely given any time to speak because Vicky continued to interrupt and talk over him as did Matt Frei, the news anchor conducting the piece.

On one such tangent, Vicky claimed it's unfair for a "straight person" to say that a "gay person" is wrong based on the paradigm of "heterosexual" marriage because that removes the hope of the "gay person" finding a "life partner."

Lively responded by saying, "It's a false premise. There is no such thing as a gay person; it's an identity you adopt."

Before he could finish, Vicky interrupted Lively once again, asking, "So you do not think people are born gay?"

While Lively responded, "Actually not," Vicky continued firing away: "So how come I can't change the way I feel? I believe God has made me the way He's made me, it's taken thirty-five years to come to terms with that, and I believe it's actually part of my God-wired identity."

At this point Lively tried to encourage her by saying, "Vicky, God has the power to help you to overcome your homosexual inclinations—"

Again Vicky interrupted, "That kind of teaching has been so damaging to me, and it damages so many people. It's one of those things that can really psychologically scar people."

The back and forth continued from there until they suddenly "ran out of time," but this portion of the interview was absolutely pertinent to our topic and is a real life example of why people fail to overcome homosexuality. Let's go back and examine every one of Vicky's statements.

Firstly, she argued in favor of embracing homosexuality because it gives her hope of finding a "life partner." She then declared people are born "gay" based on the assertion that she "can't change the way she feels," followed by the claim God made her "gay." Then she did something slick in implying it has taken thirty-five years for her to come to terms with her sexuality. Vicky Lively was only thirty-five years of age at the time of this interview. In the beginning of the piece, she made it clear she began experiencing SSA at the age of thirteen. So by her own admission she was not struggling with her sexuality for the first twelve years of her life. This contradiction seems to be an attempt to add credence to her claim that she was born "gay." In fact, everything she said was based entirely on her own experience, her own feelings, and her own beliefs. This is precisely the definition of irrationality, and yet Vicky has taken off running in the wrong direction feeling totally justified in embracing homosexuality. She even implied it is God's will for her life, claiming He has called her to assist other "gay Christians" to "come out" and to change the culture of the church.

She also claimed the Scriptures on homosexuality are open to interpretation: "There are many biblical perspectives

. . . I'm doing a PhD in Theology, there are many ways you can read the Bible."[43] Vicky later labeled herself a theologian, which is incredibly troubling because not once did she ever mention sin, morality, the biblical definition of marriage, God's parameters for marriage, lust, impure thoughts, or sexual immorality in her vigorous defense of homosexuality. Homosexuality, once again, is above all else a moral issue—it is either sinful or it is not. Only God, as the Creator and the only perfect moral agent, is able to establish which it is. To ignore this fact and focus on her feelings, to label the biblical perspective of sexuality as "damaging," and to insinuate God's commands are open to interpretation are all the results of embracing sin.

Vicky Beeching's message is not about righteousness or about living according to God's will. In referencing her "calling" to help others to embrace their homosexuality, she said:

> *If one of those teenagers could just see more people standing up and saying, "actually it's okay." You know the Bible, which I love and I've studied in depth, you know it doesn't actually say what we think it says about human sexuality, we've got a lot of it wrong. And I just hope there can be a message of hope to those young people to be who they are, to know that's okay, and that God loves them exactly the way that they are.*

These are bold truth claims for which Vicky provides no evidence or logical argument to prove. Furthermore, as many others have done, Vicky has tried to blur the distinction between salvation and God's love in an attempt to rationalize homosexuality. God loves *everyone,* including sinners; this is not in question. To insinuate that because God loves someone, they are saved from eternal destruction, however, is clearly erroneous. Regardless if we are Christians or sinners, it takes no action on our part to be the objects of God's unconditional love. In contrast, God's free gift of salvation requires us to actually accept it. We accept God's salvation by abandoning sinfulness and embracing Jesus Christ, not by embracing sinfulness and calling ourselves Christians.

Vicky expressed some strong opinions concerning God's Word, but again she offered no proof whatsoever that we got the biblical teachings on human sexuality "wrong" or they can be read in "many ways." Nor does she even broach the critical questions concerning the moral standing of homosexuality. She has adjusted God's Word to fit her own beliefs in an effort to enjoy the benefits of Christianity while embracing a sinful lifestyle at the same time. The truth is there is no compromise. Homosexuality is sinful. Christians do not practice sin, so attempting to rationalize sinfulness using God, the Bible, and Christianity is not only offensive to God, but it proves how dangerous and deceptive sin is. Sadly, Vicky Beeching has failed to overcome homosexuality because she has embraced her feelings and altered her entire worldview to align with those feelings, instead of adjusting her entire worldview to align with God. God can work a miracle of any magnitude at any time. So to assume one has no options for the future outside of homosexuality is proving either a severe lack of understanding of God, or a severe lack of faith in God.

**Summary**
We can glean a great deal from the life and choices of Vicky Beeching. It's interesting that by Vicky's own admission, her focus "for thirty-five years" was on her sexuality, and when it became too much to handle, she shifted her focus to work and music. She never once indicated that she shifted her focus entirely to God. This is a critical step that is absolutely essential to overcoming homosexuality, and it is a step that Vicky

has apparently not yet taken. In Vicky's mind, her feelings and perception hold more weight than God, truth, the Bible, and morality. This clearly is a profound mistake that results in bondage to sin instead of freedom from sin.

Before we move any further, I must point out the church must also share the blame in cases like Vicky's. Imagine if that Catholic priest had come out of the confessional booth, gave Vicky a hug, and then took the time to get to know, guide, and help her to overcome her struggles, instead of saying a prayer that had absolutely no positive effect whatsoever before dismissing her. Imagine if at that Christian conference, instead of a sea of people praying and rebuking Satan and demons in front of a crowd of thousands, if some dedicated church leaders took Vicky to a private setting, talked with her, and dedicated their time and energy into helping her, instead of sending her away worse off than when she arrived. Vicky may have actually been spared the intense struggles she faced in the coming years that slowly turned her mind toward following her feelings instead of following Christ. Nevertheless, it is not the things we have no control over that we will be held accountable for; it is the things we have absolute control over—how we live our lives and what we do with what God entrusts us with—that we will be held accountable for. In Vicky's case, instead of never wavering from the truth, never wavering from God's Word, and never ceasing to find out how to overcome sinfulness (something *every* single person on the planet must do to find God), she gave in to her feelings and hardened her heart. She began trying to explain away every challenge to her sinfulness with excuses or rationalizations such as, "That is so damaging to me and others," and that is "psychologically scarring." Of course rationalizations like these are absolutely irrelevant to the matter at hand. They are essentially implying if the truth hurts someone, then we must stop telling the truth because their comfort level is more important. Wisdom says to accept truth and reject what is false. Foolishness says to accept only what is comfortable and makes you feel good regardless if it is the truth or not. Instead of hardening our hearts and rejecting the Scripture, which is absolute truth, we need to get over our hurt feelings and accept the truth; not reject the truth in order to spare our feelings. The latter only leaves us with a lie and the problem we've had all along. Unfortunately, Vicky Beeching is only one of many who have failed to overcome homosexuality for this reason.

# Success Story

I've done a considerable amount of research on "ex-gays." I've carefully read the personal accounts describing the before, during, and after of the "homosexual" lifestyle of both men and women, but there was one that stood out to me above the others. One account of a former "lesbian" was exceptionally powerful because of how long she'd lived the "homosexual" lifestyle, how influential she was in supporting and advocating homosexuality, and how drastic she's changed since successfully overcoming homosexuality.

Charlene Cothran was brought up in the church but rejected God at age fifteen and embraced "lesbianism" at age nineteen. For nearly thirty years Charlene was not only a proud "lesbian," she was a "homosexual" activist who worked hard to promote homosexuality. For ten years, she organized massive social events and subsequently launched *Venus Magazine*—a national publication for "gays" and "lesbians" of color. Charlene amassed a tremendous following, including support from the major "LGBT" activist groups that were primarily led by wealthy Caucasian males. In partnering with Charlene, these activist groups were able to dispel the myth that homosexuality was limited by race, and because of

Charlene's huge following the "homosexual" agenda gained momentum through diversity and numbers.

Charlene was successful and made a lot of money, but after thirty years, and ten years in a committed "lesbian" relationship, she was neither happy nor content. Now, looking back, the reason is perfectly clear. In an interview with Pure Passion[44], Charlene explained: "The devil deceived me, and he deceived many thousands and thousands of others into believing that we could be happy. You know that's the deception that this is a happy life, that this is a gay life, this is a gay pride, we are happy . . . none of that is true. None of that is true."

Charlene's path out of "lesbianism" began when her mother passed away. Charlene recalled how, a few months prior, her mother told her that she never thought she'd see her again. It wasn't a reference to this life. It was a reference to the afterlife and Charlene knew it. When her mother died, Charlene was suddenly the one responsible for taking care of her ailing grandmother, and in purchasing a burial plot with three graves (one for her mother, one for her grandmother, and one for herself) she was forced to consider eternity. With her mother now in eternal glory, Charlene began to question if homosexuality was truly the lifestyle God intended for her. Was this truly the path that would lead her to happiness, and contentment, and eventually to God? She knew in her heart and from her decades of experience in the "homosexual" lifestyle that it would not. She said:

> *Facing my mortality . . . forced me to begin to think about things that are spiritual. There were times in my soul that I wanted someone to share with me how I could get out of this captivity that I was in. Certainly I had the knowledge of Christ, but I did not know that I could be free in my flesh again. I always*

*struggled with that. Can I ever be free in my
flesh? Can I ever not want a woman? Can I
ever not look at a woman and desire her? Can
I ever break free of that?*

It was during a discussion with a pastor that Charlene was
finally challenged with the truth. The pastor said, "I can see
that you want to come back to Christ. You know how to get
free, but you can't figure out how to stay free. And you feel
as though God can't use you because you've been so public
about your lesbianism. God intends to use all of that."

The conversation left Charlene speechless because it was
absolutely true. She began to cry as the solid walls of her
hardened heart began to crack and crumble. The pastor gave
Charlene two opportunities to pray with her and accept Christ,
but Charlene declined. She recalled how God spoke to her
spirit in that moment and said, "You are going to choose this
day who you're going to serve. I've been here, I've loved
you, I've protected you, I've helped you. Today is your day,
you're going to choose, and if you choose me, then I'm going
to use you, I'm going to make you so happy, and I'm going to
use all the gifts that I've developed in you for my own glory.
But if you say 'no,' if you refuse me today, then I'm going to
allow you to go on and drift off and do whatever you want,
but at the end of that road is going to be judgment. Today is
the day you will choose."

Charlene immediately began to wrestle with the implications of abandoning homosexuality. She began to question
how she could abandon her "homosexual" lifestyle, and consequently her livelihood, and still survive. She finally said,
"I don't know how I'm going to do it. All I know is that I
have to trust God in this moment, and I'm going to choose
God in this moment." It was then that the ever-persistent
pastor asked Charlene a third time if she would pray with her,
and Charlene finally agreed. So at age forty-two Charlene

made the decision to abandon homosexuality. Two weeks later, at a "gay" event she'd already committed to attending, Charlene was given the opportunity to come out again, this time as a Christian. Before a group of her peers (a panel of "gays," "lesbians," and influential publishers with whom Charlene was well acquainted) she was prepared to say whatever God wanted her to say. It wasn't easy, but when Charlene was asked about the future of her magazine she answered unashamedly:

> *The direction of* Venus *is going to change one hundred eighty degrees . . . Our mission up until now has been to encourage gays and lesbians to stand up and be who you are in the community, and come out of the closet and be proud and let your parents and neighborhoods know; we're going now in the opposite direction. We want to let gays and lesbians know that this is* not *what God intended. And* Venus *is going to now instruct people on how to get out of homosexuality, and not only that, but you can't just get out on your own, it takes a committed relationship with the Lord Jesus Christ, and this is what He's done for me.*

The entire room was shocked into silence for several moments afterward. The event finally resumed, and when it was over, Charlene was tempted to skip the reception and leave immediately to avoid any negative reactions from those in attendance. The Lord challenged her to remain and encouraged her with the fact that this was now her new ministry and the purpose that He'd given her to fulfill. Charlene thought she was in for some cold responses, but she explained how one by one people began to approach her and admit that they too were unhappy in the "homosexual" lifestyle and desired to get out of it as well. People began to thank her for being bold enough to speak the truth, particularly in that pro-homosexual setting. Suddenly it was crystal clear to Charlene that God was using individuals like her, who had actually experienced all that the "homosexual" lifestyle had to offer, to minister directly to those who are lost and held captive in that lifestyle. This is a job that people like Charlene are perfect for, and it took that incredible response for her to realize it.

> *Now these people can't look at me the same way they might look at a Baptist preacher or a Pentecostal preacher who's not walked in those shoes. They can't look at me and say, "she doesn't know what she's talking about. She's just being prejudiced against me." They know I was in the same thing that they were in; they know that I was stuck in the same flesh struggle that they were stuck in, but I am free!*

Since then Charlene has become a minister and has been used by God to change people's lives using her personal experience as proof that change is indeed possible with God. Of course, she's received the backlash and the hatred of the "tolerant" "LGBT" community who has condemned her, sent her hate mail, and accused her of being brainwashed. As a keynote speaker at an AFTA (Americans for Truth about Homosexuality) event, Charlene addressed this backlash by saying:

> *It seemed as if anyone who is bold enough to stand up and say that homosexuality is sin got added to the gay activist hate list . . . And so now that my name has been added to this hate list, I'm actually kind of proud of it, for two reasons: One, it tells me that I'm doing*

*something right. Gay activists don't waste
their time and energy. They go after people
whose ministries are effective . . . And also, if
they believe that I've been brainwashed, then
essentially they are acknowledging that there
has indeed been a change in me. Because
remember, these are people who knew me. All
of you are just taking my word for it. They
knew me. And they knew that I was a diehard
lesbian. And yet they see and know that I've
changed. And they can't attribute it to repara-
tive therapy, and they can't attribute it to anything except Jesus Christ.*[45]

We can learn a great deal from Charlene Cothran and
the path she's set in successfully overcoming homosexuality.
Not only do we see it is indeed possible to be free from the
captivity of homosexuality (even for those who have lived
a "homosexual" lifestyle for thirty years or more), but that
freedom is available to everyone who wants it and is willing
to work tirelessly for it. The truth lies in the evidence. The
evidence can be seen and heard in the lives of people like
Charlene who stand as proof of total deliverance, which
simply cannot be denied or explained away.

## Comparing and Contrasting

I've presented two real-life examples of women who both
came up in the church and both tried to overcome homosexuality. One failed; one succeeded. Let's take a look at
the reasons why. First, I will present the irrational positions
held by Vicky Beeching (which are rationalizations she actually said outright or directly implied), then I will present the

conflicting rational positions held by Charlene Cothran and many other shining examples of "ex-homosexuals."

**Irrational:** Saying, "God can help you overcome homosexuality," is damaging.

**Rational:** Saying, "God can help you overcome homosexuality," is not damaging, it is truthful. The truth of this statement is in the evidence. Charlene Cothran and many other "ex-homosexuals" have not only experienced this reality, but they have focused their ministries on helping others to overcome homosexuality based on this reality. Pointing those who struggle with homosexuality to God has not proven to be damaging but to be a beacon of hope to those who accept it. Because Vicky has yet to experience this hope and this salvation, that does not make this statement false. Nor does it explain away the countless people who have experienced God's hand in their lives and can say, "God helped *me* overcome homosexuality." These individuals are eternally grateful that God can indeed help people overcome homosexuality and would adamantly disagree with Vicky Beeching's position.

**Irrational:** God hasn't removed my "homosexual" desires; therefore, He will not or is unable to remove them.

**Rational:** That which God has yet to accomplish has no impact whatsoever on His ability or His intention to accomplish those things. We can never doubt God or assume He cannot cleanse us of any type of sinfulness once we are fully submitted to Him. Vicky continues to point out that she's thirty-five years old, and her feelings haven't changed despite praying to God to change them. This, of course, doesn't mean God cannot, or never will change them. If those feelings remain, there is a reason why, and many times it has nothing to do with God. As we will see in the coming chapters, because we ask God to do something, that doesn't mean

He has to do it when and in the method we expect Him to. Secondly, asking God to do something while we are in error does not obligate God to oblige us in any way. Thirdly, asking God to do something that is our responsibility is a mistake because while we're waiting on Him to do it, He's waiting on us to do it.

**Irrational:** I cannot change my feelings.
**Rational:** "'I can do all things through Christ who strengthens me,' (Philippians 4:13, NKJV) including changing my feelings." Vicky absolutely can change her feelings and has proven it. Before, she *felt* it was wrong to "come out" and say she was a "lesbian", but her *feelings* changed, and now she *feels* it is not only okay to do, but it is the right thing to do. This proves if Vicky truly surrenders to God and gives Him her whole heart, God will assist her in changing her feelings once again: this time to abandon her pro-homosexual agenda in favor of God's agenda.

**Irrational:** I was born "gay."
**Rational:** I've already presented plenty of evidence that proves this assertion false. No one is born "gay," but we are all born into sin and need to accept Jesus as our Lord and Savior in order to be born again and set free from sin. "I was born 'gay,'" as we have discussed, is not a factual statement; it is merely a false statement made in an attempt to mask the fact that Vicky transitioned from an individual struggling with SSA to someone who chose to stop struggling, to give in to her feelings, and build her identity on "lesbianism" because that is much easier than continuing to fight against those feelings. Saying, "I was born gay" might convince people like Vicky they are justified in embracing homosexuality, but that certainly doesn't make it true, and it certainly doesn't convince God that approving of sin and indulging in it is justified either.

**Irrational:** Biblical Scriptures on homosexuality can be read in many ways, and the Bible doesn't say what we think it says regarding human sexuality.

**Rational:** Biblical truth remains biblical truth regardless of human thought or interpretation. Therefore, the clear and consistent condemnation of homosexuality in the Bible is indeed accurate and authoritative. It's interesting to note Vicky never says she reached this conclusion *before* deciding to "come out" as a "lesbian," nor does she detail on what basis she's reached this conclusion. In any case, her assertion is plainly false and a weak attempt to undermine God's Word merely to escape conviction for violating God's Word. Vicky continuously says how much she loves the Bible, how much she's studied the Bible, and how the Bible is her favorite book, but if that was true, she would be *doing what the Bible says,* not distorting the Bible's message to condone her sinful lifestyle while leading others astray as well. Notice Vicky never explains in what ways these Scriptures (taken individually or collectively) could be read in *any* way that condones or promotes "homosexual" behavior. This is because it is impossible to make the Bible say what it doesn't say. In her debate with Scott Lively, she attempted to bolster this claim by referencing the PhD, which she had yet to actually acquire, as if to say, "Because I'm pursing a PhD, that means I'm right." It appears she wasn't ready for Lively's response informing her he actually has a PhD in theology. At this she quickly backed off by saying they could agree to disagree. She never mentioned the PhD she pursued was not in theology, ancient Greek or Hebrew, or Bible, but in technology and ethics, which she switched to Christianity and sexuality after "coming out." The point is this: pursuing a PhD doesn't make what you're saying correct, and even acquiring a PhD doesn't make what you're saying correct. Vicky can ignore the Scriptures and try to explain them away, but she cannot change what the Scriptures say. We must remember God's commandments are not cryptic, and God does not change His mind concerning sin. If "homosexual" behavior was detestable to God in the Old Testament era, and it was detestable to God in the New Testament era, then it is still detestable to Him today, and it will remain detestable to Him forever because "homosexual" behavior will *always be* a violation of God's Moral Law.

**Irrational:** God made me the way that I am.
**Rational:** Immoral conduct resulting from a predisposition does not become moral conduct as a result; nor can immoral conduct be rationalized based on that predisposition. In other words, immoral conduct remains immoral regardless of the circumstances. So when Vicky says, "God made me the way that I am," she's attempting to rationalize homosexuality but fails because this falsely implies God made her "gay," which further implies that her being "gay" is part of God's will. Again the truth is we are all born into sin and sin manifests itself in a variety of ways. God knows this and gave us the solution to cleanse ourselves of all sin through Jesus Christ, and it is God's will that we accept His free gift of salvation and live pure and godly lives every day in total submission to Christ.

**Irrational:** God loves me the way that I am.
**Rational:** God's love is not predicated on one's moral status, nor does God's love excuse one's immoral status. God loves us unconditionally. This means the statement, "God loves me the way that I am," is absolutely true. However, do not be deceived by the way this statement is often used in an attempt to justify sinful behavior. This does not mean: "Because God loves *me* the way that I am, God also loves the *way* that I am." Notice the difference? Mankind is the object of God's love, not man's behavior. God does not love homosexuality, which is abundantly clear, so this true statement used in a deceptive

fashion does absolutely nothing to change God's position on sinful behavior. As previously stated, it is not God's will that anyone of us remain bound to sin, especially when Christ suffered and died for us so we could be free from sin.

**Irrational:** "Living a lie" is wrong, so it's okay to be who you are.

**Rational:** A creation's identity is not established by their predisposition or behavior; a creation's identity is established by their Creator. Anything outside of this is living a lie. This whole idea that struggling with SSA equates to "living a lie," and "coming out" as a "homosexual" equates to "being who you are" is a fallacy. This is how the false reasoning goes: "I experience SSA. To deny my feelings is to deny who I truly am and to live a lie, which is wrong. To accept and embrace my feelings is to accept and embrace who I truly am and to live honestly, which is right. Therefore, to do what is honest and right, I must adopt the 'homosexual' moniker and embrace homosexuality." The truth is a private struggle with SSA is not "living a lie." It is an honest struggle against sinfulness, which deep down we all know is wrong—this is precisely why it's a struggle. Despite what Vicky says, it is not okay to give in to sinfulness no matter what it is or what the circumstances are. Sinfulness separates mankind from God, so regardless how strong our feelings, urges, and temptations are, if they are sinful we are obligated to fight against them without ceasing because our eyes are fixed on God, not sinfulness.

**Irrational:** Denying I am "gay" eliminates any hope of ever finding true love.

**Rational:** True love is found in God. Any "love" that is not grounded in God is not true love. The dream of true love is one that most people share. Nevertheless, regardless how much we might desire to find true love in another person, that desire cannot supersede our love for God. Our love for God is proven in our actions and our obedience to God's Word, so to assume denying one's "homosexual" disposition precludes the possibility of true love is firstly not necessarily true, but secondly it is a sinful desire. So in using this argument to rationalize homosexuality, Vicky has proven her top priority is not God and His will, but her love life, which is essentially idolatry. Secondly, Vicky is not all-knowing and therefore cannot possibly dictate what can and cannot happen in her future. Once people seek God first and wholeheartedly there is no telling how God will bless them. Yes some "ex-gays" do remain single and celibate indefinitely, but other "ex-gays" (including people I personally know) have found true love and are now happily married and have children with their spouses. Once again, this concept is not unique to those struggling with homosexuality. People like me who have yet to find a spouse can't use that as an excuse to lead a sexually sinful lifestyle in pursuit of true love. As I prepared myself for the likely possibility I'll never get married (which means I will never experience sex), someone struggling with homosexuality must come to the same place of total and complete submission to God's Moral Law in this and every other area. Love is selfless not selfish.

**Irrational:** I feel God has called me to help change the church to be pro-homosexual.
**Rational:** God created every single person with a distinct purpose for him or her to fulfill in life. That purpose is never to lead a sinful lifestyle, nor is it to teach others how to live a sinful lifestyle. Vicky couldn't be any more out of order here. She feels that God called her to encourage others to "come out" and enter a world she herself hasn't even lived for any significant length of time. Considering this, how can she possibly know for a fact that it is good and godly? Vicky would do well to talk to someone like Charlene Cothran who has

lived the "homosexual" lifestyle for three decades and find out if it's something God wants His church to embrace and practice. Vicky is not only way off the mark with this assertion, which is once again based off of her feelings, but she is missing God's true calling for her life. Notice she didn't say it was her calling to help lead people toward *God;* she feels her calling is to help lead people toward *homosexuality.* This is dangerous and abhorrent.

In contrast, Charlene Cothran knows what God has called her to do, and she's been doing it ever since she gave her whole heart to God and overcame homosexuality in the process. She's been a shining light to countless people in the "homosexual" community and to the body of Christ as a whole. She's dedicated her unique experience, talents, and influence to help people out of homosexuality by leading them to God. So the question we must ask is, would God really call Vicky to lead people *into* homosexuality and call Charlene Cothran to lead people *out* of homosexuality? Clearly the answer is "no." These are conflicting callings; if both are true, there's a contradiction and God never contradicts Himself. Clearly, Vicky Beeching is mistaken because her perceived calling doesn't align with God's Word at all. I personally believe God has a plan for Vicky that would see her successfully overcome homosexuality and then use her fame, talents, experience, and influence to change countless lives by showing others how to come out of homosexuality instead of how to embrace it. Vicky has a free will to reject God, however, so until she decides to change her feelings and put God first, she will never fulfill her God-given purpose.

## Conclusion

It is possible for everyone who identifies as "gay" to overcome homosexuality. The fact that many try and fail does not change this fact. The distinction between those who fail and those who overcome homosexuality is clear. Those who try to adjust God's Word to suit their sinfulness instead of acknowledging and purging their sinfulness to obey God's Word will never find success. The state of deception and denial is a dangerous place to live, and yet there are many who profess to be Christians who find themselves there. Vicky Beeching isn't alone. She is following the detrimental path of those like "gay Christian" Matthew Vines who insists that homosexuality is morally acceptable if they are committed loving relationships. Those open to deception like Vicky, Matthew, and Pastor Chris, along with countless others who profess Christianity, should be acutely aware of the prison of deception in which they've locked themselves. 1 Corinthians 6:9 cannot be any clearer in warning us: "Do not be deceived," it begins, "Neither the sexually immoral nor idolaters nor adulterers nor male prostitutes nor homosexual offenders . . . will inherit the kingdom of God." Anyone who tries to use Scripture to contradict this absolute truth is deceived, and no one who is deceived and unrepentant will succeed in overcoming homosexuality.

# 9

# Troubleshooting Homosexuality

Life is inundated with problems, and troubleshooting is an invaluable process for solving life's problems. The problem-solving process begins with effective troubleshooting, and effective troubleshooting is predicated on an effective troubleshooter. For example, when we have computer problems, we call an IT specialist for help. Based on the information we provide, the IT specialist then takes a systematic approach to solving the problem. This is called troubleshooting, and if it's done correctly, the process will establish the root problem, which will then determine the appropriate solution, and in the end the problem will be solved. What's important to note here is that the reason this process works is because the IT specialist has already been trained extensively to troubleshoot and solve computer problems. They are already intimately familiar with the hardware and software of computer systems and how they relate to each other. Without this knowledge they would be as clueless as we nontechnical folk are in solving these problems. Thankfully, because they are trained experts they are uniquely qualified to be a troubleshooter.

This is imperative because in order for us to accurately troubleshoot homosexuality, we must become experts ourselves. We must also possess the knowledge necessary to effectively identify and solve the problems related to homosexuality. We've already thoroughly analyzed the natural aspect of homosexuality, but in order to gain a full understanding of the issue, we must now thoroughly analyze the spiritual aspect as well. Just like computer software is contingent upon computer hardware, in life the natural is contingent upon the spiritual—the former cannot function without the latter. Therefore, we will proceed by looking below the surface of homosexuality to become intimately familiar with the spiritual side of the matter.

This requires analyzing what I call the Adam Effect. The Adam Effect is a simple model I designed to clearly show what transpires spiritually regarding morality and immorality. This fundamental principal will be the foundation on which everything that follows is built. Further, understanding the Adam Effect and its three components will streamline the process of troubleshooting homosexuality to determine the proper solution.

# THE ADAM EFFECT

The Adam Effect is so named because it illustrates the spiritual reality of mankind, which directly resulted from Adam's sin in the Garden of Eden. The simple version of the Adam Effect is a model that is easy to understand because it only includes three components and illustrates the relationships between those components. The three components of the Adam Effect are the heart, the sinful nature, and the Spirit. We will begin to analyze this model by defining what each component is, how it functions, and what its purpose is before detailing the characteristics of the relationships between them.

# The Heart

*Definition:* the core and essence of a human being.

The heart is the primary component of the Adam Effect. The heart is the core of a person, and who they truly are. It's the center and the most significant facet of a human being. Just as natural DNA is absolutely vital for life and totally unique to each individual, the heart defines and identifies every human being in the most complete and accurate way. Out of the heart flow one's thoughts, will, and motives. In other words, it is the source of what we think, what we do, and it is the reason *why* we do what we do. This is precisely why the heart is so significant in the Bible. It is mentioned over eight hundred times and we are repeatedly admonished to love, obey, trust, seek, serve, and trust the Lord with all of our hearts. With this understanding it becomes perfectly clear we're commanded to do these things with the entirety of our core and our essence, with the entirely of our thoughts, our will, and our motives for a purpose. The primary objective of the heart, the reason it was created, was to love, see, hear, feel, know, and obey God. It was fashioned to be permanently connected to God and prepared to be used by God whenever and however He sees fit. However, because of Adam's sin, our hearts are naturally sinful as they are enslaved to the sinful nature by default.

# The Sinful Nature

*Definition:* the regenerative living evil inherent in every human being.

The sinful nature is essentially a spiritual parasite in that it benefits from its host (the heart) to the detriment of its host. The sinful nature is the heart's nemesis; it is the part of humans that is naturally immoral, that naturally opposes God, and relentlessly craves and feeds on sinfulness.

The Apostle Paul, who was the most influential person in the New Testament next to Christ, struggled with his sinful nature exactly like every one of us. He detailed his struggle with overcoming sin in the book of Romans saying:

"I know that nothing good lives in me, that is, in my sinful nature. For I have the desire to do what is good, but I cannot carry it out. For what I do is not the good I want to do; no, the evil I do not want to do-this I keep on doing. Now if I do what I do not want to do, it is no longer I who do it, but it is sin living in me that does it. So I find this law at work: When I want to do good, evil is right there with me. For in my inner being I delight in God's law; but I see another law at work in the members of my body, waging war against the law of my mind making me a prisoner of the law of sin at work within my members" (Romans 7:18–23).

In this several things are made quite clear that must be kept in mind as we explore this issue:

- There is nothing good in the sinful nature.
- The sinful nature works to prevent us from carrying out the good we know to do.
- Sin living within us can and will enslave us.
- Evil is ever present when the sinful nature is alive and well.
- The sinful nature wages war against the mind and the body.

The sinful nature operates primarily through deception, persuasion, and oppression. It communicates directly to you exclusively through your own thoughts, and it accomplishes its goals through your feelings, desires, and urges. Because the sinful nature is a part of you, it knows exactly how to use your thoughts, experiences, and proclivities to entice you into a sinful lifestyle that would see you relinquish your control and allow the sinful nature to control you. Below are some of the primary ways in which the sinful nature functions.

- It perverts morality.
- It exalts pleasure above God.
- It glamorizes sinfulness to distract from godliness.
- It fosters irrationality and folly.
- It numbs the feeling of guilt to rationalize sinfulness.
- It prevents the divine purpose from being fulfilled.

The primary goal of the sinful nature is murder. This spiritual parasite demands to be constantly fed, which strengthens it until it finally kills its host. This means your sinful nature's entire strategy is to systematically kill you without you ever realizing it. Satan is not your number one enemy nor are demons your number one enemy. Your number one enemy is your sinful nature. It is with you wherever you go and it is relentless in its desire to kill you through the incessant indulgence of sin. There is a pattern set when the heart is enslaved by the sinful nature. There are specific and inevitable consequences that lead to a singular destination, which is eternal destruction. Make no mistake about it, the sinful nature is entirely evil and cannot be appeased at any time under any circumstances.

## The Spirit

*Definition:* the third person of the trinity; God.
The Bible refers to the Spirit in many ways: Holy Spirit, Spirit of God, Spirit of Jesus, Spirit of Christ, Spirit of truth, the Counselor, Spirit of sonship, and the Spirit of the Lord to name a few, but these are all references to one and the same Spirit. The Spirit is first of all a person not a force, and secondly that

person is God. The Spirit is God and God is the Spirit. Paul tells us plainly: "Now the Lord is the Spirit, and where the Spirit of the Lord is, there is freedom" (2 Corinthians 2:17). This is spectacular news for those who make the wise decision to serve the Spirit instead of the sinful nature, because when the Spirit dwells within the heart there is literally freedom inside of us.

As opposed to the sinful nature that pushes, forces, urges, lies to us, hurts us, and numbs us to the guilt of sin, the Spirit leads, prompts, and encourages. He speaks the truth to us, helps us, and convicts us of sin. Because the Spirit is literally God inside us, we have the great benefit of the all-powerful, all-knowing, universal Creator working within us to aid us in whatever we do. This means that even when we are alone, we are never truly alone.

The primary objective of the Spirit is to express unconditional love through a personal relationship with the object of that love: mankind. In order to have a personal relationship with mankind of the highest quality, God chose to be as close to mankind as possible. This is why, of all places for God to inhabit, He chose to literally take up residence inside the heart of man. Just as there is a pattern set when the heart is enslaved to the sinful nature, there is also a pattern set when the heart is enslaved to the Spirit. There are specific and inevitable consequences that lead to a singular destination, which is eternal life.

## The Pure and the Impure Heart

The heart is a slave by nature. It cannot function on its own; it functions through total devotion and obedience to its master, which is either the sinful nature or the Spirit. The master of the heart not only controls the heart, but it is actually a part of the heart. Thus the heart is essentially an incomplete container or vessel that is driven by one of two captains toward one of two eternal destinations. This means there are only two possible conditions of the heart: impure and pure. The impure heart is empty, hardened, and dying because it is enslaved to the sinful nature. The pure heart is full, moldable, and thriving because it is enslaved to the Spirit. Let's closer examine both of these states.

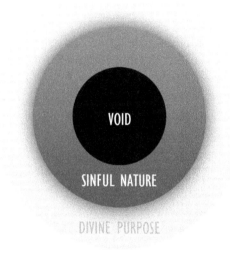

**FIGURE 4**
The Impure Heart

### The Impure Heart

As a result of sin, the heart is a malfunctioning vessel from its inception. It is impure, it is opposed to God, and consequently it becomes hardened and eventually immutable. The image of the impure heart (Figure 4) is a representation of what all of our hearts look like from birth.

At the center of the heart you see there is a big void. This is due to the fact that we are all born spiritually incomplete. The problems that result are monumental because that feeling of emptiness and incompleteness drives people to try to fill that void themselves, but in the end they are still left empty and incomplete because the task is impossible for us. People trying filling it by having unbridled promiscuous sex, abusing drugs and alcohol, chasing after money and possessions, and seeking thrills, but nothing they try is enough to fill the void. This is why, the rich and the famous (people we think are happy because they have everything they want), wind up in rehabilitation centers, mental health facilities, hospitals, and jail. What's worse, many even wind up committing suicide. It is a horrible experience to feel that void at the center of your being, and it's an even worse experience trying and failing to fill that void.

Beyond the void is the sinful nature. It is a part of a person's core and essence from birth and as you can see in the image it is alive and active from the beginning. It grows as we grow and the more we feed it by sinning the more powerful it becomes and the closer to death we get.

Finally, the specific divine purpose is also a part of a person's core and essence from birth. Notice, however, that while the void and the sinful nature are active in the impure heart, the specific divine purpose is dormant. This is because it is absolutely impossible to fulfill one's divine purpose with an impure heart that is enslaved to the sinful nature.

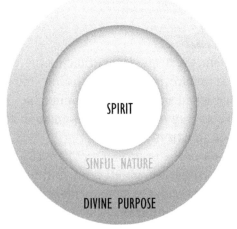

**FIGURE 5**
The Pure Heart

## *The Pure Heart*

When functioning properly the heart is totally receptive to God and perceptive of God; it is sensitive and completely open to be shaped and molded by God. Notice that in the image of the pure heart (Figure 5), instead of the void at the center of the heart, there resides the Holy Spirit. The Holy Spirit is the *only* one who can fill that void and until the heart is enslaved to the Spirit, the void will remain. The Holy Spirit of God is absolutely invaluable, not simply because He fills the emptiness that nothing else can fill within us, but He leads, guides, and helps us through life. When we are confused He brings clarity, when we are about to fall into sin, He warns us. When we sin He convicts us so that we will repent and be washed clean. When we do what is right and pleasing to God, He blesses us. When the Spirit is the master of the heart, the fruit of the Spirit flows from the heart and manifests in our lives: "love, joy, peace, patience, kindness, goodness, faithfulness, gentleness, and self-control" (Galatians 5:22–23).

Notice when the Spirit is master of the heart, the sinful nature is not only no longer in control, but it is rendered dormant. It is important to understand the sinful nature doesn't magically disappear because as long as we live in these corruptible bodies it will always be possible for us to sin. Through Christ we have redemption and by the Spirit we are taught how to please God and abstain from sin.

Finally you see now the specific divine purpose is no longer dormant. It is only by the Spirit that we are each able to realize and fulfill our individual divine purposes, which is the reason God made us and gave us life.

# The Relationships Between the Three Components

The relationships between the three components of the Adam Effect actually mirror a triangle that we are all quite familiar with: the love triangle. A love triangle is a relationship involving three people. Most often the central person in the triangle is romantically in love with two people. Those two people are both in love with the central person. If they are aware of one another they often absolutely despise one another. This is precisely what we find in the Adam Effect (Figure 6). Here the heart mirrors the central person in the love triangle; the sinful nature and the Spirit are the opposing forces that the heart must choose between.

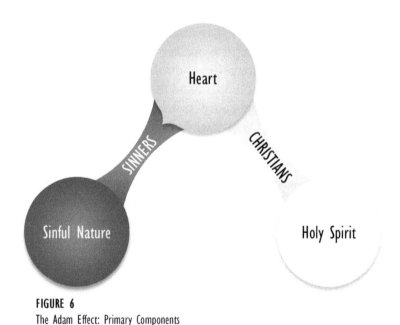

**FIGURE 6**
The Adam Effect: Primary Components

**The Heart and the Sinful Nature**
This relationship is based entirely on sinfulness. Sin is the fuel that keeps it alive. Here the heart is a slave to a master that is utterly evil. Consequently, while the sinful nature continues to be fed, it increases in power and influence while the heart weakens and deteriorates. The Defining characteristics of the heart/sinful nature relationship are as follows:

- Involuntary—this relationship is entered into automatically without prior consent.
- Enduring—this relationship is impossible for the sinful nature or the heart to sever.
- Reciprocal—as the heart feeds the sinful nature by doing evil, the sinful nature stores up evil inside the heart.
- Exclusively Beneficial—despite the illusions, only the sinful nature benefits from this relationship
- Entirely Negative—the longer the relationship endures the more the heart suffers; the bigger the void grows until the inevitable conclusion of eternal destruction is reached.

**The Heart and the Spirit**
This relationship is based entirely on love. Pure, unconditional, reciprocal love is the fuel that keeps it alive and prospering. Here the heart is a slave to a Master who is utterly good. Consequently, the heart is purified and cured of the weight and captivity of sin. There are several consequences of this relationship: God's will is done for and through each of His children, each one of God's children is able to fulfill his or her God-given purpose, each one is saved from the sinful nature and eternal destruction, and each one is guaranteed eternal life in heaven with God. The defining characteristics of the heart/Spirit relationship are as follows:
- Voluntary—this relationship is entered into by choice.

- Enduring—this relationship, when entered properly, lasts forever.
- Reciprocal—as the heart feeds the Spirit the Spirit lavishes blessings upon the heart.
- Mutually Beneficial—both the heart and the Spirit are enriched in increasing measures as this relationship continues.
- Entirely Positive—the longer this relationship endures the more the heart thrives; it is complete, functioning properly, and flourishing until the inevitable conclusion of eternal life is reached.

### The Spirit and the Sinful Nature

Like the relationship between light and darkness, it is impossible for the Spirit and the sinful nature to be active and in control at the same time. There is no compromising, no synergy, and no compatibility between the two. They are always at odds, as good and evil are at odds. The only thing they have in common is the desire to rule the hearts of man.

# The Adam Effect Model

The extended version of the Adam Effect (Figure 7) essentially illustrates the two roads that Jesus spoke of: the narrow road that leads to heaven traveled by few, and the broad road that leads to destruction traveled by many. On the left side you can see the inevitable progression of the heart/sinful nature relationship, which is the path of the sinner:

1. The sinful nature produces evil desires.
2. Evil desires lead to sin.
3. Sin leads to death.
4. Sinful death results in eternal destruction.

# The Adam Effect

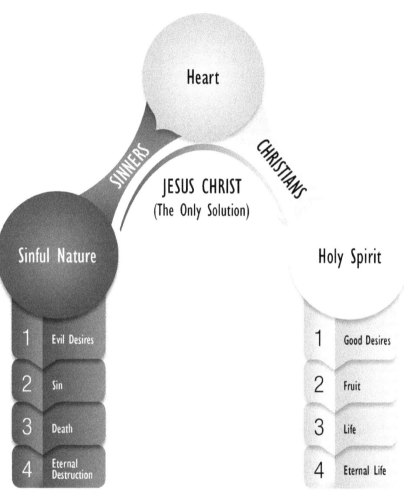

**FIGURE 7**
The Adam Effect: Full Model

On the right side you can see the inevitable progression of the heart/Spirit relationship, which is the path of Christians:

1. The Spirit inspires good desires.
2. Good desires produce the fruit of the Spirit.
3. Righteousness leads to abundant life.
4. Abundant life leads to eternal life.

# How to Troubleshoot Homosexuality

Now that you understand the nature and relationships between the three components of the Adam Effect, your crash course on the spiritual reality of mankind is complete. With this foundation set you are now fully equipped to select any specific sin, troubleshoot it using the Adam Effect as a backdrop, and determine the proper solution to eliminate the root of the problem and all the resulting sin-related problems. Troubleshooting requires three general steps:

1. Identify the root of the problem.
2. Establish the proper solution to the problem.
3. Implement the proper solution to the problem.

### 1. Identifying the Root of the Problem

What happens when we run the sin of homosexuality against the Adam Effect? Where does homosexuality fit in the scheme of things? Remember the progression detailed in the extended version of the model when the heart is enslaved to the sinful nature:

1. The sinful nature produces evil desires.
2. Evil desires lead to sin.
3. Sin leads to death.
4. Sinful death results in eternal destruction.

We've established homosexuality is indeed sinful, so homosexuality naturally fits in the second stage of the progression: evil desires lead to sin. Notice how far removed this stage is from the actual root of the problem and also how close this stage is to the two ultimate stages: death and eternal destruction. Now it is perfectly clear that praying for God to remove one's "homosexual" disposition is an ineffective solution on its own because it fails to address the root of the problem. The third stage of the progression reveals the symptoms, the *acts* of the sinful nature, which flow from the root of the problem. So what are the acts of the sinful nature?

> The acts of the sinful nature are obvious: sexual immorality, impurity and debauchery, idolatry and witchcraft; hatred, discord, jealousy, fits of rage, selfish ambition, dissentions, factions and envy; drunkenness, orgies and the like. I warn you, as I did before, that those who live like this will not inherit the kingdom of God (Galatians 5:19–21).

The first sinful act on the list is sexual immorality, the category that homosexuality falls into, and with the possible exception of witchcraft, every remaining sinful act on this list is a component of homosexuality. This is a powerful indication of just how dangerous homosexuality is. In order to prevent that which inevitably follows homosexuality, we must do some backtracking. Walking backward through the progression, we can see homosexuality is preceded by evil desires, and evil desires are the product of the sinful nature. We can glean three invaluable lessons from this. Firstly, homosexuality (as well as any other sinful addiction/lifestyle) is a direct result of the sinful nature. Secondly, the heart enslaved by the sinful nature is impure, as it is filled with evil, which results in sinfulness. Thirdly, the mind (which is one of the fundamental elements of the heart) is fixed on the desires of the sinful nature when the heart is impure.

> Those who live according to the sinful nature have their minds set on what the sinful nature desires; but those who live in accordance with the Spirit have their minds set on what the Spirit desires. The mind of sinful man is death, but the mind controlled by the Spirit is life and peace; the sinful mind is hostile to God. It does not submit to God's law, nor can it do so. Those controlled by the sinful nature cannot please God (Romans 8:5–8).

This illuminates the core issues of homosexuality and yet this is foreign to most people who make the critical error of assuming homosexuality is the root of the problem. Homosexuality is not the *root* of the problem; it is a *symptom* of the root of the problem. Because this symptom is a problem in itself, it is often mistaken as the sole issue. We cannot afford to duplicate that error. The root of the problem is the sinful nature.

## 2. Establish the Proper Solutions to the Problem

What we've seen is a root of the problem, which is spiritual and manifests in many ways. It produces an array of problems that ultimately manifest in natural reality. This implies the solution to homosexuality is not singular but pluralistic: partly spiritual and partly natural. Since the spiritual aspect is paramount, we will begin there. If the root of the problem is the sinful nature, which makes it impossible to submit to God's law and leads inevitably to death and eternal destruction, then the solution would be to overcome the sinful nature, purify the heart, and set the mind on the Spirit, which leads to life and peace.

The heart must be freed from the bondage of the sinful nature (the wrong master) and become totally subservient to the Spirit (the right Master), which ultimately leads to eternal life. How is this transition made? What is the solution to the root of the problem, i.e., the sinful nature? The answer is Jesus Christ. This is precisely the conclusion the Apostle Paul came to after detailing his personal struggle with sin in the book of Romans. He said, "What a wretched man I am. Who will rescue me from this body of death? Thanks be to God—through Jesus Christ our Lord" (Romans 7:24–25). In other words, there is but one solution to overcoming the sinful nature, and that is the Lord Jesus Christ who God the Father sent for that purpose. This is why when a sinner makes the wise decision to accept Jesus as their Lord and Savior, part of their prayer is, "Lord Jesus come into my heart." This is the first step of the transition and, once Jesus Christ enters the impure heart, He purifies it. He is the *only one* who can purify the heart. The Spirit then enters the clean place and fills the gaping void as only He can. It is only through Jesus Christ that we receive the gift of the Spirit. Jesus promised the Holy Spirit, saying:

> If you love me, you will obey what I command. And I will ask the Father, and he will give you another Counselor to be with you forever—the Spirit of truth. The world cannot accept him, because it neither sees him nor knows him. But you know him, for he lives with you and will be in you . . . All this I have spoken while still with you. But the Counselor, the Holy Spirit, whom the Father will send in my name, will teach you all things and will remind you of everything I have said to you. Peace I leave with you; my peace I give you (John 14:15–17, 25–27).

As you can see, once we allow Christ to be the Lord of our lives, and prove our love to Him by keeping His commandments, He does what we are powerless to do ourselves. He breaks the chains that bind our hearts to the sinful nature, purifies our hearts, and fills the emptiness with the Spirit of God. On top of all this, Jesus leaves us with peace as well, which is absolutely invaluable. So essentially, upon accepting Jesus Christ, our hearts are completely transformed from impure, empty, hardened, and dying, to pure, filled, moldable, and thriving. This is the critical part of the solution that many people only mentally assent to, but don't actually commit to and fulfill.

This transition is not something one merely tries out, nor is there any jumping back and forth from one path to the other because Christianity and practicing sin are lifestyles—totally conflicting lifestyles. One is a moral lifestyle; the other is an immoral lifestyle. When done correctly the transition from the sinful lifestyle to the Godly lifestyle is permanent, and the proof of that change is reflected in the moral conduct of the individual who made the transition. Just as there is no bouncing back and forth between these two extremes, there is no such thing as a middle ground. As previously established, due to the objectivity of morality, we are either moral or immoral. Anything less than godliness is ungodliness; therefore, the illusion of a middle ground is actually enslavement to the sinful nature in disguise. There are many people, I know some personally, who prayed for Jesus to come into their hearts. They renounced their sinful lifestyles and pledged their lives to Jesus as their Lord and Savior with tears and conviction, and everyone rejoiced and welcomed them into the family of Christ. Beyond that, absolutely nothing changed. Despite the prayers that were prayed and the tears that were shed, these people went right back to the sinful lifestyles that they publicly renounced. The fact is that those who accept Christ into their hearts and then continue to sin have not truly accepted Christ into their hearts. This critical step is not about saying some words, shedding some tears, and making an effort to do more good than bad; this is a fundamental change that completely transforms the heart, mind, and spirit of a person. There is no going backward after this step because only one master will be served and that master, the rightful master, is the Spirit. This is about becoming an entirely new creation, entirely different from before. "Therefore, if anyone is in Christ, he is a new creation; the old has gone, the new has come" (1 Corinthians 5:17). The difference is loving God with one hundred percent of one's heart (i.e., the entirety of their core and essence, their thoughts, will, and motives). Even ninety-nine percent or anything less is simply not enough.

The proof of this transition is detailed in Scripture:

> You, however, are controlled not by the sinful nature but by the Spirit, if the Spirit of God lives in you. And if anyone does not have the Spirit of Christ, he does not belong to Christ. But if Christ is in you, your body is dead because of sin, yet your spirit is alive because of righteousness. And if the Spirit of him who raised Jesus from the dead is living in you, he who raised Christ from the dead will also give you life in your mortal bodies through his Spirit, who lives in you (Romans 8:9–11).

In fact, the Bible makes it abundantly clear that those whose hearts are slaves to the sinful nature are children of the devil, and those whose hearts are slaves to the Spirit are children of God, heirs to God's throne, and co-heirs with Christ. Jesus Christ is the difference.

> No one who lives in him keeps on sinning. No one who continues to sin has either seen him

or known him. He who does what is sinful is of the devil because the devil has been sinning from the beginning . . . No one who is born of God will continue to sin, because God's seed remains in him; he cannot go on sinning, because he has been born of God. This is how we know who the children of God are and who the children of the devil are: Anyone who does not do what is right is not a child of God; nor is anyone who does not love his brother (1 John 3:6, 8–10).

So as we can see, the primary solution is Jesus Christ, the indwelling of the Holy Spirit is a direct result of accepting Christ as Lord and Savior, and in submitting to the Holy Spirit one hundred percent, the proper foundation is set to overcome homosexuality and combat all the residual problems associated with homosexuality.

### 3. Implement the Proper Solutions to the Problem

Homosexuality is a lifestyle, which means overcoming homosexuality requires a lifestyle change. So what does that lifestyle change require? In troubleshooting homosexuality we've thoroughly examined the issue, and against the backdrop of the Adam Effect, it has become clear the array of consequential problems is not limited to the natural. The root of the problem (the sinful nature) is spiritual, and it is the *symptoms* or *outworkings* of that problem that are natural. The principal issue is the sinful nature doesn't miraculously disappear when someone dedicates their life to Christ and receives the Holy Spirit. That fundamental transition is the beginning—there is much work to be done afterward. In the next two chapters I will detail how to implement the proper solutions to successfully overcome homosexuality.

# 10

## "The Dos" for Overcoming Homosexuality

While it was imperative to establish the sinfulness of homosexuality, particularly to quell the controversy and debates surrounding the issue, that is not the sole purpose of this book. If Christians truly wish to help people, we cannot simply go around identifying problems; we must also offer solutions to those problems. Establishing a problem exists is merely the beginning of a process. We must now continue the process by offering help, hope, and solutions to those in need. So if you are personally struggling with homosexuality, or if you're one of the many who know and love individuals living a "homosexual" lifestyle, what follows will be of great benefit to you and to anyone you are led by the Spirit to help with this issue.

While homosexuality is a complex issue with an array of causes that impact each individual uniquely, I believe it is possible for every single person who experiences SSA and/or identifies as a "homosexual" to overcome homosexuality.

The path to victory is not an easy one, but it surely isn't an impossible one. The process I've laid out here includes a total of fourteen steps divided between this chapter and the next. Here the focus is on the seven things one absolutely *must* do to overcome homosexuality.

## 1. Give God Your Whole Heart

I cannot possibly overemphasize how critical this step is. This is the foundation upon which all the other steps are fixed, so to skip this step or fail to complete it is to guarantee failure. The reason for this has already been established in our analysis of the Adam Effect, but in addition to that there is an abundance of actual evidence to prove this is true. I've studied numerous accounts of people who successfully overcame homosexuality after years of struggling with it. In examining the journeys of these "ex-homosexuals" I discovered a common element. Despite the variety of backgrounds (some were atheists, some abandoned Christianity, others were Christians struggling with trying to please God and live as "homosexuals" at the same time), these "ex-homosexuals" all came to the *same resolution*, the same turning point that led them to freedom from homosexuality. After years of "trying everything" and failing, these ladies and gentlemen took a step back for a moment and realized their true problem was inside their hearts. Although they all came to the conclusion God was the only solution to their troubles, it suddenly occurred to them that they had failed in two significant ways in seeking God to repair their lives. The first was in their objective (the *reason* for seeking God), and the second was their execution (the *way* in which they sought God). After a completely honest and objective evaluation, it became clear their objective in seeking God was to get something from Him. They turned to God hoping He would rid them of their "homosexual" disposition. They discovered the error in this approach was they essentially attempted to use God by seeking Him with an ulterior motive. In addition, as we've established in the previous chapter, they eventually discovered homosexuality was not the root of their problem anyway. Regarding the failure in execution, whether consciously or unconsciously, they all realized they never truly and fully submitted to God. They never gave God their *whole* heart; they'd merely given Him part or most of their hearts. At some point they all came to this realization: *Even submitting ninety-nine percent to God and giving Him ninety-nine percent of my heart is not enough. Until I am willing to submit to God one hundred percent and to give Him one hundred percent of my heart, I will continue to fail in life, and my struggle with homosexuality will never end.* It is absolutely imperative that anyone who is struggling to overcome homosexuality reaches this same conclusion. Sadly, those who fail to overcome homosexuality do so because they fail to take this step. They either maintain a hard heart by not fully submitting to God, or they merely mentally assent to submitting to God, while in reality they are reserving a portion of their heart for sin. In the past, the goal for many homosexuals was to figure out how to love God and receive all of His benefits, and love homosexuality at the same time. The problem is this never works because the two are totally incompatible. It is impossible to love both; you will always love one and hate the other. Luke 16:13 makes this principle quite clear: "No servant can serve two masters. Either he will hate the one and love the other, or he will be devoted to the one and despise the other." What's more, the Bible repeatedly commands us to fear the Lord. While this is often misinterpreted as a command to be afraid of God, this is not at all what God commands of us. Proverbs 8:13 makes this clear: "The fear of the LORD is to hate evil." We've already established that homosexuality is evil, which means that you can no longer love it. To overcome homosexuality you must learn to hate it, and in doing so you prove your love for God. Remember this is an all or nothing situation. God requires your whole heart and He deserves it.

Those who are still secretly in love with homosexuality resist this step and start making excuses. In their heart they say things like, "I'll obey God as long as I understand everything first and it feels like the right thing for me to do," "I'll obey God as long as I agree with His commands," and "I'll obey God as long as things in my life are going well." Those in this position are telling God that they don't love Him unconditionally, and they're proving they still haven't offered God their whole heart. God loves us unconditionally, and until we reciprocate that unconditional love, we will never be free from sin.

"What exactly does giving God my whole heart mean?" you might ask. It means a transition must be made from doing life your way to doing life God's way. There is no fifty-fifty split; there is no compromise or negotiation of any kind. It is either one hundred percent God's way, or nothing. So to anyone who has yet to fully submit to God, make a vow that from this moment forward you will agree with God and completely obey Him regardless of the circumstances, regardless of what you think, feel, like, and/or understand. Offer yourself as a living sacrifice to God, dedicating your entire life to Him in total submission, including everything you own, recognizing nothing belongs to you—you are simply a steward over what God has entrusted to your care. Again, you don't even belong to yourself. You belong to God who purchased you at the price of His own Son. This is not a temporary thing, this is not something you plan to try out or test for a week or a month; this is a permanent life decision. You can't love God part-time. Not when He loves you full-time. So instead of the lifestyle you've practiced all this time, which says, "Let *my* will be done," adopt a new and better lifestyle, which says to God as Jesus did, "Yet not my will but *yours* be done" (Luke 22:42).

In addition, seek God *for God,* not for anything you want *from God.* Many people have tried everything they can think of to escape the clutches of homosexuality but failed, and they look to God as a last resort. They say, "Fine, God, I'll seek you now. Free me of homosexuality," and are surprised and thoroughly disappointed when nothing happens. The problem is not that God is unable or unwilling to help; the problem is in the seeking. To seek God with any ulterior motive is sinful. So regardless of your history with Christianity, dedicate (or rededicate) your life to God by truly accepting Jesus Christ into your heart and seek God as an automatic response to His unconditional love with no ulterior motives.

Submission and obedience are automatic responses to God's unconditional love. God already loves you unconditionally—He loved you before He ever created you, but once you love God the right way, that love for God will manifest itself not in words alone, but in actions. Your life, what you do, what you say, and what you think will all change to conform to God's Word out of submission and obedience to Him. You will experience victory when you are able to honestly say, "It doesn't matter what I think or how I feel. What matters is what God said and what God knows. God is always good, and He's always right, so regardless of what I think or feel, whatever He commands me to do, I'll do, and whatever He commands me to not do, I won't do. I am led by the Spirit, not by my sinful nature."

Once you reach this place of absolute humility and obedience, when your true goal is to seek God in order to find God, then you will find Him, and your life will change forever. Then you will be aligned with God's will and be able to fulfill your God-given purpose. God Himself said:

> "For I know the plans I have for you," declares
> the Lord, "plans to prosper you and not to
> harm you, plans to give you hope and a future.

Then you will call upon me and come and
pray to me, and I will listen to you. You will
seek me and you will find me when you seek
me with all of your heart. I will be found by
you" (Jeremiah 29:11–14).

Notice God will not be found until you seek Him with
*all* of your heart. Remember also that according to Jesus, the
greatest and most important commandment is: "Love the Lord
your God with all your heart and with all your soul and with
all your mind and with all your strength" (Mark 12:30). This
is how you give God your whole heart (again the entirety of
your core and essence, your thoughts, will, and motives). Until
this step is fully executed in the right way, failure is eminent.

Consider the words of Charlene Cothran describing
her personal experience in successfully overcoming
homosexuality.

*I stand as evidence that the Holy Spirit can
and will change you if you give God your
whole heart. When you pray, pray that God
will come into your whole heart and change
your whole heart, not just to take the gay thing
away, not just to take the lesbian thing away.
It doesn't work like that. You have to give God
all of you. He's changed many things in my
life, not just the lesbianism; I had an anger
problem. He's had to break that up. [There
are] so many things that we have in our lives
that have to be turned over, all of us. Give
God your whole heart and He'll put you back
together again.*

So to those who are struggling to overcome homosexuality, you can't keep riding the merry-go-round of life and

think something will change and you'll experience something new that'll suddenly end your struggle. Surrender everything that you have and everything that you are. Be totally submitted to God in every area of your life. Then God will change what you can't and bless you with the power and victory over homosexuality.

## 2. Purify Your Mind

This step, which is invariably linked to the previous, involves two components: mindset and thought life. We find this connection between submission to God and the mindset in Romans 12:1–2.

> Therefore, I urge you, brothers, in view of God's mercy, to offer your bodies as living sacrifices, holy and pleasing to God—this is your spiritual act of worship. Do not conform any longer to the pattern of this world, but be transformed by the renewing of your mind. Then you will be able to test and approve what God's will is—his good, pleasing, and perfect will.

A person simply cannot take their old sinful mindset into the newness of Christ and be fully submitted to God. It's utterly impossible. The pattern of this world embraces, practices, promotes, and defends sinfulness. Before Christ, this was the pattern you conformed to. After Christ, as your spirit was recreated, your mind must be renewed, and you must conform to God's pattern instead. Remember, what the mind is set upon determines the fate of the individual.

> Those who live according to the sinful nature have their minds set on what that nature desires; but those who live in accordance

with the Spirit have their minds set on what the Spirit desires. The mind of sinful man is death, but the mind controlled by the Spirit is life and peace; the sinful mind is hostile to God. It does not submit to God's law, nor can it do so. Those controlled by the sinful nature cannot please God (Romans 8:5–8).

Those who successfully overcome homosexuality change their mindset. Their minds are no longer fixed on their sinful nature, the source of "homosexual" desires; it is fixed on the Spirit and the Spirit's desires. This is the difference between death on one end of the spectrum, and life and peace on the other.

The second component of purifying your mind is your thought life. Fully submitting to God requires you to submit your thought life to Him as well. This entails entertaining pure thoughts instead of impure thoughts. The trouble is many people believe there's nothing wrong with entertaining whatever thoughts come to their minds — as long as they don't physically do anything wrong, they assume they haven't done anything wrong. Their motto is, "There's no harm in thinking it." This couldn't be further from the truth. Thoughts are absolutely harmful because thoughts inspire words and eventually actions. Remember, sin starts in the mind, and thoughts are the primary tool the sinful nature uses to communicate with you and entice you to sin. Therefore, it is indeed harmful to entertain sinful thoughts.

Controlling one's thought life is not only absolutely essential in overcoming homosexuality, but it's something many people don't even know is possible. The common misconception is we have no control over our thoughts, which results in the erroneous notion: "There's nothing wrong with thinking whatever comes to my mind because I have no choice in the matter." This is obviously false and is proven false by the fact that we all have thoughts that cause powerful negative effects that we avoid at all costs. There are things in life that disgust us, enrage us, make us sad or terribly uncomfortable, and whenever thoughts of those things enter our minds, we quickly dismiss them to avoid those inevitable negative effects. This proves we do indeed have control over our minds; we all have the capacity to reject thoughts we shouldn't entertain. Not only do we all have this wonderful ability to control our thought lives, as Christians, we are *obligated* to control our thought lives.

We have been given the power through Christ to control the contents of our minds so we are able to love the Lord God with *all* of our minds as the Scripture commands. Remember: erotic thoughts left unchecked lead to erotic actions, so in order to prevent erotic actions one must prevent erotic thoughts. How is this done? The Apostle Paul explains our ability to accomplish this in his description of our spiritual weapons.

> The weapons we fight with are not the weapons of the world. On the contrary, they have divine power to demolish strongholds. We demolish arguments and every pretention that sets itself up against the knowledge of God, and we take captive every thought to make it obedient to Christ (2 Corinthians 10:4–5).

This is excellent news for us. We are powerless on our own, but through Christ we have the power to demolish the strongholds in our lives. The "homosexual" disposition is a stronghold that can be demolished with our spiritual weapons like any other stronghold over our minds. *Having* divine weapons, though, isn't enough. It is our responsibility to *use* our divine weapons effectively to win the battle over our minds. We must remain diligent because, as you are well aware, evil thoughts can pop into your mind at any moment of the day or night. When you identify the thought as evil, you have two options: cast it out of your mind immediately, or allow it to play out. Obviously, the right choice is to cast the thought out of your mind immediately. However, you can't stop there. Once you cast an evil thought out of your mind, you can't continue to think about not thinking about that thought. Why not? Because you'll eventually wind up still thinking that thought. To prevent this you not only have to *stop* thinking the evil thought, you must *start* thinking a good thought instead.

So what constitutes a good thought? Good and acceptable thoughts are described in Scripture: "Whatever is true, whatever is noble, whatever is right, whatever is pure, whatever is lovely, whatever is admirable—if anything is excellent or praiseworthy—think about such things" (Philippians 4:8). Now be careful. Someone might argue that based on this Scripture, there is nothing wrong with thinking about a certain person they find to be lovely. Do not fall into this trap. Good thoughts won't violate any of these requirements, so if thoughts of an individual you find to be lovely lead to impure thoughts, then that obviously violates this Scripture, and you need to stop thinking about that individual. The Apostle Paul makes it plain and clear. He says, "Clothe yourself with the Lord Jesus Christ, and do not think about how to gratify the desires of the sinful nature" (Romans 13:14). No one knows better than you what your sinful nature desires, so this means you are also intimately aware of what thoughts you should not be entertaining.

This definitely takes practice but commit to this and stay committed to it. The moment you start giving in to your thoughts is the moment you start relinquishing your self-control to your sinful nature, and before you know it, your thoughts will become so powerful that they'll result in the actions you're trying to avoid. In addition to this, you have to change what you feed yourself. Monitor what you allow into your heart in order to keep your heart pure. The results of a truly purified mind are pure speech and pure actions. This is precisely what all of us need, this is precisely what God requires, and anyone struggling with homosexuality must commit to this in order to overcome homosexuality.

### 3. Devote Yourself to Prayer

What is prayer? Prayer is quite simply communicating with God. Prayer is important because you need God more than you can fathom. You need to know Him, you need His guidance and direction; in short, you need to be in a strong relationship with God.

Why should you pray? Effective communication is essential in building strong relationships, and prayer, done correctly, is effective communication with God. Too often people want the benefits of a good relationship with God (blessings, healing, favor, protection, etc.) before ever establishing a good relationship with God. It doesn't work like that. Prayer is a key element in the equation. The relationship between you and God is the most important relationship you'll ever have, and if that relationship is going to be good, there must be effective communication. This is what prayer facilitates. Prayer is also essential for spiritual well-being. "Air is to the natural man as prayer is to the spiritual man," is a common phrase that accurately expresses the vital nature of prayer. Humans can't survive long naturally without air; likewise, humans cannot survive long spiritually without prayer.

When should you pray? As often as possible. It doesn't have to be an hour-long discussion, but you should acknowledge God in everything you do. "In all your ways acknowledge him, and he will make your paths straight" (Proverbs 3:6). You should start every day in prayer, and you should end every night with prayer. A common mistake is to believe God is too busy to listen, or He can only hear prayers that are eloquent and perfectly communicated. Both of these notions are false. As God's child you can pray to Him at any moment, and He will hear you. The instant you gave God your whole heart, He gave you that right. The Bible says, "Be joyful always; pray continually; give thanks in all circumstances, for this is God's will for you in Christ Jesus" (1 Thessalonians 5:16–18). In other words, pray to God without hesitation whenever and as often as you please. God is not too busy. On the contrary, He's waiting to hear from you.

How should you pray? Firstly, you must prepare yourself for prayer, otherwise you will get distracted and your prayers will be ineffective. 1 Peter 4:7 says, "Therefore be clear minded and self-controlled so that you can pray." Give God your undivided attention. Then you can pray to God effectively through your words, your thoughts, and/or the Spirit. All three of these are quite simple. When you pray through words, you talk to God as easily as you talk to anyone else. It is easier to pray to God through your thoughts because God knows your thoughts and the contents of your heart. So when you are unable to speak out loud, you can still communicate effectively to God through your heart and mind. The wonderful thing about the Spirit is He intercedes for us. There are times when you need to pray but don't know how to put your prayer into words or thoughts. In these times we are not without hope. The Spirit inside us understands exactly what we need and He communicates to God the Father on our behalf.

What should you pray for? It's normal to pray to God for help, healing, favor, protection, blessings, desires, etc. As someone struggling with homosexuality, your prayer should primarily be for God to help you to learn how to love Him and prove your love for Him by keeping His commands. You should be praying for God to open your heart and mind so you can hear His voice and understand His Word. You should be praying for God to show you how to be more like Jesus every single day, to keep your mind and body pure and abstain from sin in every area. Hebrews 4:15 tells us Jesus was tempted in every way and yet He did not sin. If He was able to resist sin, then you have that same power through Jesus Christ who is in you. You need God's help in order to access that power every day. You should be praying for God to show you how to love yourself and how to love your neighbor the way He commanded us to. You should be praying for God's will to be done in your life, for God to show you what your purpose is, and how to fulfill it. It's also important to recognize God is not a divine combination of a genie and a lawyer—He doesn't exist only to grant your wishes and to get you out of trouble every time you call on Him. Respect Him as your heavenly Father and dedicate time to doing nothing but thanking God for His countless blessings, instead of constantly rattling off your wish list during prayer time.

While the heart of your prayer time can be focused on you, the entirety of your prayer time shouldn't be. Don't make the mistake of being selfish in prayer. The Bible tells us to "pray in the Spirit on all occasions with all kinds of prayers and requests. With this in mind, be alert and always keep on praying for all the saints" (Ephesians 6:18). If you don't take the time to pray for anyone else, then you're praying selfishly, and that is not God's desire. Praying for one another is how we help and strengthen one another. In addition to praying for others within the body of Christ, you should pray for those outside the body of Christ as well. As you struggled with homosexuality and are now finding the way out, pray for others who are still struggling. Pray diligently for those in the "LGBT" community and others caught in sinful lifestyles who desperately need salvation but don't realize it.

In good relationships effective communication is never one-way; it is always two-way. It is the same with prayer. Prayer is part communicating to God, and part God communicating to you. God speaks to us through our thoughts if our minds are controlled by the Spirit. It's our responsibility to know when it is God speaking to us and when it is our sinful nature speaking to us. This is the part where most people falter. They either never stop talking to listen to God, or they don't know God's voice well enough to identify it as God speaking instead of their sinful nature. This results in confusing their own thoughts and those of their sinful nature with God's voice, which always leads to catastrophe. This is why you often hear people say, "God told me..." followed by something totally contrary to God's Word, and yet they wholeheartedly believe what they're saying is truly from God. If you've purified your mind and submitted wholeheartedly to God's Word, you won't find yourself mistaking evil thoughts for God's voice in your prayer time. The more you hear God's voice in your heart, the more you feel the peace of His instruction and experience the blessing that comes from obedience. It will then become easier to dismiss the thoughts of your deceitful sinful nature, which wants you to believe that its sinful thoughts are actually God speaking to you. This is why it is imperative that you know God's voice.

Jesus said His sheep know His voice and follow His voice as He leads them.

> The watchman opens the gate for him, and the sheep listen to his voice. He calls his own sheep by name and leads them out. When he has brought out all his own, he goes on ahead of them, and his sheep follow him because they know his voice. But they will never follow a stranger; in fact, they will run away from him because they do not recognize a stranger's voice (John 10:3–5).

You want to know Jesus, and you want Jesus to know you by name. Those who know the voice of God are not confused by the voices of strangers. What's more, once you know what God has already said, you'll be able to discern when God speaks to your heart through the Holy Spirit inside you. God never contradicts himself, and He will never command you to do something that violates Scripture. If you've truly given God your whole heart, purified your mind, and committed to praying regularly, then it will be difficult to err by mistaking sinful thoughts and desires for God's voice. Successful Christians successfully master prayer and consequently successfully master their sinful nature and overcome sinful lifestyles.

## 4. Submit Wholeheartedly to the Word of God
The Word of God is essential to spiritual well-being. Spiritual well-being is essential to overcoming the sinful nature. Overcoming the sinful nature is essential to overcoming homosexuality. Therefore, the Word of God is essential in overcoming homosexuality. If "air is to the natural man as prayer is to the spiritual man," then food is to the natural man as the Word of God is to the spiritual man. Jesus said, "Man does not live on bread alone but on every word that comes from God" (Matthew 4:4). The spiritual man cannot be sustained on prayer alone. He needs to be fed and fed regularly.

The Word of God is Scripture, which we have today in the form of the Bible, and the Bible is invaluable because it serves so many purposes. "All Scripture is God-breathed and is useful for teaching, rebuking, correcting and training in righteousness, so that the man of God may be thoroughly equipped for every good work" (2 Timothy 3:16–17). We are all obligated to know God, please God, overcome sin, be thoroughly equipped for every good work, and fulfill our individual God-given purpose, and yet all of these things are impossible to achieve without the Bible.

If God's children are obligated to keep God's commandments, and God's commandments are collected in the Bible, how then can we possibly keep God's commandments if we don't know what they are? How can we know what they are without reading the Bible? Obviously we can't. The secrets to life, the keys to overcoming the sinful nature and homosexuality are all found in God's Word. Yet the power of the Bible is largely underestimated, neglected, or rejected altogether. This cannot be for anyone who seeks to overcome homosexuality or any other sinful lifestyle.

Regardless of your level of familiarity with the Bible (whether you grew up in the church and know the Bible well, or you spent decades rejecting the Bible and refusing to read it because you disliked and disagreed with what it says), recognize the authoritative nature of the Bible and wholeheartedly submit to that authority. A shift must be made from irrational to rational. So drop your defenses that you've built up all this time. Stop being angry because the Bible doesn't support homosexuality. Humble yourself and be thankful God loved you and cared enough for you to leave you clear instructions. The Bible is like a detailed map that shows you how to successfully navigate through this life and how to get to eternal life successfully. You do not know the way to eternal life, nor can you figure it out on your own. It takes wholehearted submission and consistent studying, absorbing, and application of God's Word to find the abundant life here on earth and to reach eternal life with God in heaven. Remember you don't know it all; God does, so even if you don't understand the reasons for God's commandments in Scripture, you're still obligated to obey those commandments. Even if you dislike God's commandments or feel you know a better way of life, you're mistaken and you're still obligated to obey God's commandments.

I must stress the fact that the Bible is no ordinary book. So to sit and read it as you would a novel or a magazine is a mistake. The Bible contains the words of eternal life, it is alive and consequently can't be read and its contents absorbed in one sitting. This is why Christians spend their lives studying God's Word, and even those who've read the Bible from cover to cover multiple times still don't know or understand it all yet. When you submit to God's Word and commit to studying it regularly, you open up the doors of your heart. You allow God to fill you up with His truth, which allows you to keep your mind pure, your spirit strong, and your sinful nature defeated. The Bible says:

> Blessed is the man who does not walk in the counsel of the wicked or stand in the way of sinners or sit in the seat of mockers. But his delight is in the law of the Lord, and on his law he meditates day and night. He is like a tree planted by streams of water, which yields its fruit in season and whose leaf does not wither. Whatever he does prospers (Psalm 1:1–4).

Notice the delight and focus of the man or woman who is blessed is not on sin but on God's Word. Notice also it was not in the *reading* of God's Word that the blessing came. It was through the *meditation* on God's Word day and night that the blessing came. This is a key principle even seasoned Christians often overlook. Do not make this mistake.

Now remember the Bible isn't only used for teaching, but for rebuking and correcting. This is the part people don't like because it challenges them to their core and forces them to consider how they're living and where they will spend eternity. At this point those who aren't fully submitted to God's Word start hardening their hearts again, instead of letting God's Word rebuke and correct them as necessary. They get defensive and decide to either reject the Bible altogether, or they start to pick and choose which Scriptures they'll agree with and obey, and which ones they won't based on their feelings and opinions. This obviously does not fit into this process of fully submitting to God by giving Him your whole heart and dedicating your whole mind to Him. Just as we cannot approach God conditionally, we cannot approach the Word of God conditionally either. This means if the Bible says something you don't like, you recognize the problem is not with the Bible; it is with you. If the Bible says something you don't agree with, the problem is not with the Bible, it is with you.

The Scripture likens the process of rebuking and correcting to pruning a plant in order to help it flourish. Being pruned isn't fun. Being disciplined doesn't feel good. Being convicted hurts. Yet God's Word does all these things to us because these are all things we need in order to flourish. The purpose of God's Word isn't to make us feel good; it's to tell us the truth, to reveal God to us so that we can know Him instead of knowing *about* Him.

Consider the words of the psalmist and note his passion and admiration for God's Word:

> How can a young man keep his way pure? By living according to your word. I seek you with all my heart; do not let me stray from your commands. I have hidden your word in my heart that I might not sin against you. Praise be to you, O Lord; teach me your decrees. With my lips I recount all the laws that come from your mouth. I rejoice in following your statutes as one rejoices in great riches. I meditate on your precepts and consider your ways. I delight in your decrees; I will not neglect your word (Psalm 119:9–16).

The theme here is consistent with the previous Scripture: reverence for God's Word, meditation on God's Word, delight in God's Word, and wholehearted submission to God's Word.

When you reach this place of love, appreciation and total submission to God's Word, your life will inevitably change, and your focus will no longer be fixed on homosexuality—it will be fixed on Jesus Christ. So don't underestimate, neglect, or reject God's Word anymore. Instead, value it and embrace it. This means all the doubt and the ill feelings you've carried in the past for the Bible and Christianity must all be erased. You can't doubt God's Word and hope to obey God's Word. So instead of fighting the Bible, trying to find loopholes in it, and trying to interpret it in ways that excuse sin, fully submit to it and do what it commands you to do. You can no longer ignore the Scriptures that condemn homosexuality. Instead, embrace those Scriptures, be thankful for those Scriptures, and commit to applying the truth of those Scriptures to your life through unwavering obedience. This is how you submit wholeheartedly to God's Word.

Finally, part of submitting to God's Word is the commitment to studying God's Word. You must study the Bible with more fervor than you've studied anything in your life. Of course, this requires time and dedication, but this is not only essential; it is worth it. You'll discover the Bible is like your best friend. The more you read and understand the Bible, the more enriched your life will become. So commit to studying the Bible at least once a day. Apply what you learn to your life. Pray for understanding with the portions you find difficult. Consult a Bible-teaching pastor, Christian friends, and family members for clarity, and discuss the Word of God regularly. The more of God's Word you fill yourself with, the easier it will be to maintain your purity and the less you will be inclined to sin. The less you're inclined to sin, the easier it will be to overcome homosexuality.

## 5. Die Daily

Jesus first introduced the task of dying daily when He set the requirements for being Christians. "If anyone would come after me, he must deny himself and take up his cross daily and follow me" (Luke 9:23). To emphasize the severity of this, Jesus also said, "Anyone who does not carry his cross and follow me cannot be my disciple" (Luke 14:27). So what is the significance of taking up one's cross? Yes, this was a foreshadowing of the fate Jesus and many of His disciples would face in being crucified, but it was also a parallel to what must be done spiritually inside the hearts of every individual who decides to follow the pattern Christ set for life. Understanding this parallel requires an understanding of crucifixion. Crucifixion was a popular form of execution in ancient Rome. It was a torturous, gruesome, humiliating, and effective form of capital punishment. Roman citizens were exempt from being tortured and executed in this fashion, but crucifixion was specifically reserved for the slaves and aliens who were the worst criminals. The convicted criminals were beaten, scourged, and forced to carry the heavy beam of their cross all the way outside the city to the place of execution. There they were hung on a cross and crucified unto death. This was a drastic means of purification. Not only were the criminal undesirables eradicated from the city of Rome, but also the gruesome nature of their execution incited fear in an effort to keep others from breaking the law and suffering the same fate. This is the key to understanding Jesus' message, because this is exactly how the sinful nature relates to us. The sinful nature is alien to mankind (it was never part of God's perfect design), and it is the worst criminal because it is guilty of attempted murder. Do not forget the sinful nature has a singular objective: to do evil to and through you in an effort to kill you. Therefore, the sinful nature must be eradicated with extreme prejudice like those who were convicted to suffer death by crucifixion in ancient Rome. Carrying the cross was a precursor to this gruesome death. Jesus' instruction was to do this daily. So what does that mean for us today? There were three components to the command: "deny himself, take up his cross daily, and follow me." This translates to self-denial, self-sacrifice, and complete obedience. Self-denial means you must say "no" to the sinful nature's urges and pleadings every single day. Self-sacrifice means you are not only fully prepared to suffer and die for Christ, but you sacrifice your old sinful lifestyle and your sinful nature every single day. Complete obedience means whatever God commands, you obey without question or hesitation regardless of the circumstances every single day.

This theme of dying daily and crucifying the sinful nature is carried all throughout the New Testament. "Those who belong to Christ Jesus have crucified the sinful nature with its passions and desires" (Galatians 5:24). Remember, the antithesis of this is that those who do *not* belong to Christ Jesus have *not* crucified the sinful nature with its passions and desires. So the question is not whether or not you say you belong to Jesus—the question is, what have you done with your sinful nature? The truth determines your position in Christ, and if you haven't crucified your sinful nature, there is no possible way that you can overcome homosexuality or any other sinful lifestyle.

We learn how we are to deal with the sinful nature in the book of Romans:

> For we know that our old self was crucified with him so that the body of sin might be done away with, that we should no longer be slaves to sin—because anyone who has died has been freed from sin. In the same way, count yourselves dead to sin but alive to God in Christ. Therefore do not let sin reign in your mortal body so that you obey its evil desires. Do not offer the parts of your body to sin, as instruments of wickedness, but rather offer yourselves to God, as those who have been

brought from death to life; and offer the parts of your body to him as instruments of righteousness" (Romans 6:6–7, 11–13).

This is a detailed description of what it means to die daily. It also bolsters Jesus' message, which is essentially: "unless you crucify your sinful nature, keep it dead, and obey me, you are not a Christian and eternal life does not belong to you."

Never ever forget who your most dangerous enemy is. It's not Satan; it's not demons; it's your sinful nature. Your sinful nature remains with you wherever you go and is one hundred percent dedicated to killing you. If you've seen any classic horror franchise, you're well aware the villain dies at the end of the movie but always comes back somehow to start killing all over again in the sequels. Your sinful nature is the exact same way. It's resilient, it's relentless, and it's a scavenger. Defeating it on Monday doesn't mean you won't revive it on Tuesday. Understanding this is critical to putting it under and keeping it under every single day. If your sinful nature is powerful, it's because you fed it and allowed it to become powerful. If your sinful nature is defeated, it's because you stood your ground and defeated it. The choice is yours. You must be even more relentless in killing your sinful nature than it is in killing you, because in the relationship between you and your sinful nature, there will always be one master and one slave. If you don't master your sinful nature, it will master you, and you'll be a slave to it all over again.

How exactly do you crucify the sinful nature? Once you dedicate your life to Christ, purify your mind, and wholeheartedly submit to God and His Word, Christ Jesus is free to purify your heart and invite the Holy Spirit to reign within you. Again, this doesn't magically make your sinful nature disappear, but in this process you are no longer a slave to your sinful nature; it no longer has power over you. From that moment on, it is your responsibility to crucify the sinful

nature by not feeding it. Anything that is sinful and anything that leads to what is sinful feeds your sinful nature,
and feeding your sinful nature breathes new life into it. Once
you revive it, it reclaims the power and control it once had
over you. The sinful nature feeds on sin no matter how small
it may seem to you, and it needs you to feed it in order for it
to survive. It is your responsibility to learn what feeds your
sinful nature and then cut all of those things out of your life.
Simply looking at a sexual image, or listening to an explicit
conversation can spark the flame of sin. Just as you have the
power to control your mind and refuse to entertain any sinful
thoughts, you also have the power to choose righteousness
instead of sinfulness every single day. Even if it's a gray
area—something you're not certain whether or not it will lead
to sin, err on the side of righteousness. Go above and beyond
to remain pure instead of taking chances.

Why must you die daily? Because you have free will, you
are a constant receptor, and you're still morally accountable
for your actions. Free will means you are not forced to be
righteous. Every day you have millions of choices available
to you, and at any point you can choose to follow Jesus or
follow your innate desire to sin. As a constant receptor you
are consistently affected by your sensory experience: what
you see, feel, hear, etc. As a constant receptor you have a
decision to make whenever you are exposed to anything that
is impure or sinful. You have to choose if you're going to
repel everything impure to remain pure, or if you're going to
give in and choose to be sinful once again. It is your sinful
nature's job to convince you to do the latter. You are in a
daily war against your sinful nature, and the instant you stop
fighting to remain righteous you give in to unrighteousness.
Moral accountability means God holds us accountable for
every thought we entertain, every word we speak, and every
action we take. So never underestimate the significance of
your choices, and never forget whom you're dealing with.

Your sinful nature is not your friend; it is your bitter enemy. The sinful nature will relentlessly hound you and constantly plead with you to appease it even in the smallest of ways. It'll tell you that you've been good long enough. It will encourage you to take a little break and have some fun. It'll promise you that God will understand and you don't have to worry about finding yourself back in the chains of your old sinful lifestyle. You can never give in to these lies. You are responsible for denying your sinful nature without exception. Remember, if it was the root of your problem to begin with, and you suffered so much while enslaved to it with nothing to look forward to but death and eternal destruction, why on earth would you compromise and go back into the slavery from which you were finally set free? Constantly keep this in mind, and stay sober about the fact that you are in a daily war for your life and your salvation.

**6. Dispel the Myths**
If you've identified as "homosexual" and lived that lifestyle for any significant length of time, you've been taught a great deal of wrong. A major part of the healing process involves unlearning what you've learned and then learning the actual truth. This requires you to dispel the myths, adopt the truth, and stand on that truth in order to overcome homosexuality. Many of the common "LGBT" and advocate myths are as follows:

- "Homosexual" and "heterosexual" are valid terms.
- There is such thing as "sexual orientation" and everyone has one.
- "Sexual orientation" determines your "sexual identity" which determines your sexual behavior.
- Experiencing SSA is equivalent to being "homosexual."
- It's impossible for true "homosexuals" to change their "sexual orientation."

- People are born "gay."
- "Homosexuals" have no control over their attractions, and therefore they have no control over their sexual practices.
- Sexual conduct is moral as long as it is consensual.
- Seeking to change your inborn "homosexual orientation" causes psychological damage.
- Identity is based on sexuality.
- Anyone who successfully abandons homosexuality was never truly a "homosexual"; they were simply living a "homosexual" lifestyle.
- Abandoning the "homosexual" lifestyle is to betray the "LGBT" community in favor of being a hateful, intolerant, bigot.
- There is such a thing as "marriage equality."
- Same-sex partners are equally efficient at raising children as opposite-sex partners.
- Gender is a fluid concept, "sexual orientation" is fixed, and neither is immoral.
- Life is supposed to be struggle free, so if you face struggles you can't overcome, your options are to either stop living or to give in and embrace your feelings.

This is by no means an exhaustive list, but you get the idea. We've previously refuted these myths with facts, and at this point you should be fully capable of distinguishing between the myths and the truth about homosexuality. The truth is the "homosexual" lifestyle is built upon a mountain of lies in an attempt to rationalize sinfulness and keep people bound in a prison of sinfulness. In order to break free and remain free from that prison, you must abandon the foundation of lies upon which you once stood; you must know the truth and stand firm on the truth. Once again we find this principle in Scripture, and it is tied directly to Christianity and to freedom. Jesus said, "If you hold to my teaching, you are really my disciples. Then you will know the truth and the truth will set you free" (John 8:31–32). This means those who don't hold to Christ's teaching are not His disciples, they do not know the truth, and therefore they are not free—they are still slaves to sin. Those who fit into this category, those whose lifestyle is founded upon lies, often don't realize the severity of their predicament. Jesus also said, "You belong to your father, the devil, and you want to carry out your father's desire. He was a murderer from the beginning, not holding to the truth, for there is no truth in him. When he lies, he speaks his native language, for he is a liar and the Father of lies" (John 8:44). The distinction is clear. You either hold to the truth and carry out God's desires, or you hold to lies, and carry out Satan's desires. There is no middle ground here, as there is no middle ground between right and wrong, godliness and ungodliness, righteousness and unrighteousness, Christ and Satan, Christians and sinners.

Jesus said, "I am the way the truth and the life. No one comes to the Father except through me" (John 14:6). The pathway to God the Father is truth in Christ, and the core theme of this entire book has been to express the truth about homosexuality. Now that you know the truth, you must embrace that truth and apply it to your life in order to experience the freedom that Christ promised.

### 7. Ask for Help

If you're like me, then you hate asking for help. I'd much rather help someone else than ask someone for help. Although it makes me terribly uncomfortable, from time to time I need help, and if I don't ask I won't get the help I need. We all need help from time to time. Refusing to ask for help when we need it is foolish, as it leaves us helpless. Understand this is a pivotal moment in your life and getting help may not only save your life, but save you from eternal damnation as well. This is something most of us don't think about while we're caught up in a sinful lifestyle. This life is not all there is, and there are only two places to spend eternity. The "homosexual" lifestyle leads to the place where no one truly wants to go, so if it takes asking for help to keep from going there, then it is absolutely worth it. The good news is there are plenty of options available to help people overcome homosexuality. There are organizations specifically dedicated to helping people struggling with homosexuality, there are pastors and counselors who specialize in this area, and there are "ex-homosexuals" who have written books and have websites and blogs where you can get help and reach out to them for assistance. Do some serious research, pray and ask God which path would be best for you to take, and then take it. All the while keep in mind countless "ex-gays" exist, and if they were able to overcome homosexuality, then you can too.

# 11

# "The Don'ts" for Overcoming Homosexuality

As there are specific things one must do to overcome homosexuality, there are specific things that one must not do to overcome homosexuality. Success cannot be had without adhering to both parts of the process. What follows are the seven things that absolutely must not be done in order to successfully overcome homosexuality.

## 1. Don't Accept a False Homosexual Identity

I recently had a conversation with a woman who is struggling to overcome homosexuality. She's a Christian who loves God and has had a difficult life. She began by saying, "I am a lesbian," and then explained her struggle to me without ever realizing the critical error she made. There are many people who are in the exact same position and make the same error, which impedes their success. It is imperative to dismantle this false perception of identity from the outset. The idea that "what I feel, I am, and what I've done, I will always be" is simply not true. Understand what your true identity is, where it comes from, and what it is founded on, and then embrace and profess that true identity. As established from the beginning of this book, a person's identity is not defined by "sexual orientation." God does not view mankind as a mix of "heterosexuals" and "homosexuals." He views us as male and female the way He created us. The whole concept of "sexual orientation" and "sexual identity" is unfounded. Once again, mankind invented the concept of "sexual orientation," the terms "lesbian," "gay," "bisexual," and all the other terms on the ever-increasing list of "sexual identities." Remember, "sexual orientation" is a modern concept that is not based on fact or science in any way. It is an abstraction, a figment of the imagination. It is absent from Scripture because this concept has no bearing on Scripture. Again, any reference to homosexuality in Scripture pointed to *behavior* not a *state of being*. In other words, the Bible never condemns "homosexuals" but acts of homosexuality. The distinction is important and is in no way an indication that we have no control over our behavior.

Further proof that the concept of "sexual identity" is false is the fact that "ex-gays" have been ostracized and attacked by "homosexual" activists for abandoning homosexuality. Why would this consistently take place? Could it be because the militant "LGBT" activists don't want to acknowledge that their ideology is entirely false? Absolutely. Those that don't attack "ex-homosexuals" instead opt for disparagement to deny "ex-gays" by saying things such as, "Well, that just proves they weren't 'gay' in the first place," or, "They're just living a lie—they're still 'gay.' They're in denial." This is not only baseless, offensive, and entirely false, it is totally contrary to the "gay rights" ideology that preaches love, tolerance, and anti-discrimination. Thankfully, there are plenty of "ex-gays" who have done us all a favor by standing tall and sharing their stories with the world. They continue to prove it is possible to overcome homosexuality and acknowledge their true identity in the process. You can do the exact same thing. Though you may have adopted this ideology and built your entire identity on homosexuality, come to terms with the fact that such identities are false. "Sexual orientation" doesn't determine one's identity, nor does it give anyone moral license to act on sinful feelings, urges, and attractions. If that were the case, everyone would be free to have sex without boundaries and justify it because it's just a result of their "sexual orientation." After all, if this is the justification "homosexuals" use, why can't it be extended to other "sexual orientations"? Pedophiles and the incestuous are now using this exact same argument in an attempt to justify their behavior, and more will undoubtedly follow. This, however, is obviously illogical and sinful.

Keep in mind that nobody can tell you who you are because they don't have enough knowledge to do so. In fact, even when you are uncertain about your identity, God isn't. He's the only one qualified to show you who you are and what your purpose is in life. You did not create yourself, and therefore you cannot look within yourself to establish your true identity. "Sexual orientation" didn't create you, so you cannot look to "sexual orientation" to establish your true identity. Your true identity is established by God and God alone, the one who created you in His image with specific gifts and talents to fulfill a specific purpose. So even if you're still struggling with homosexuality, break the mentality of an identity based on homosexuality. Stop referring to yourself as "gay," "lesbian," "bisexual," or "homosexual." Stop perpetrating the labels society has adopted. Instead, start identifying yourself as a man or a woman, a child of God, and a Christian. This is your true identity because this is the way God sees you. Remember, God is always right, so if you are a male Christian, God sees you as a son, which means you are indeed a son of God and a brother of Christ. If you are a female Christian, God sees you as a daughter, which means you are indeed a daughter of God and a sister of Christ.

Now, I am well aware of how complex this step can be. I fully understand the severity of the implication here: for those who have built their identities upon homosexuality and expressed that identity for years, abandoning that identity could be viewed as essentially abandoning one's self. This immediately begs the question, "Who am I then?" which could clearly be frightening. Do not worry. The only one who is capable of answering that question has been waiting for you to seek Him so that He can give you the answer. You're not alone in asking, "Who am I?" I believe every human who has yet to connect with his or her Creator has pondered this same question of identity. Remember your identity is based on and determined by the Creator. Any identity that has excluded the Creator is a false identity. Anyone who is struggling with homosexuality cannot cling to a false "homosexual" identity and successfully overcome that false "homosexual" identity. So see yourself as the person God sees, because the person God sees is who you truly are: a Christian man and a son, or a Christian woman and daughter, not a "homosexual."

## 2. Don't Pray Ineffectively

The importance of devoting your life to prayer was stressed in the previous chapter. Here the focus is on avoiding a fruitless prayer life. This is important because it is possible to be fully devoted to prayer and yet continually pray amiss. As you've already seen, and perhaps already experienced, praying earnestly for the wrong thing and/or in the wrong way yields no answer from God. We've all had prayers go unanswered, but we must remember the problem is *never* with God; the problem is *always* with us. In our fast-paced society we've trained ourselves to satisfy our desires as fast as possible because waiting is torturous. As a result we suffer from impatience. To accommodate this, we've deceived ourselves into believing God works on our timeframe instead of on His timeframe. When we pray we want God to answer immediately, and if not we become terribly irritated and begin to question God and His commandments as if there is some fault to be found there. As a result of this impatience and frustration, many people simply give up their quest for righteousness. They seek God, limit Him to their timeframe, and when they don't see any results, they give up and go right back to their problem instead of relentlessly seeking the solution to their problem. They say things such as, "I tried praying but God didn't answer me." This is folly born of ignorance and impatience. First of all, to not receive the answers we seek doesn't mean God has not heard our prayers or He's not in the process of answering our prayers. God's timing and His method are both perfect; our timing and our methods are not. Understanding this requires faith and patience, qualities which you need to acquire and maintain.

Secondly, there are conditions that must be met in order for God to hear and answer prayers. If those conditions aren't met those prayers will go unheard and unanswered. These are the three basic contributing factors to unanswered prayers: unrighteousness, timing, and God's will. Salvation from homosexuality is definitely God's will, so if that prayer has yet to be unanswered for you, then it is either due to an unrighteous condition (you remain guilty of some sin that you need to repent for and be cleansed of), or it is a matter of timing (God is working on it and will finish it in His time not yours.)

Unrighteousness is a prayer deterrent. It is utterly impossible to be unrighteous and have an effective prayer life. On the contrary, "The prayer of a righteous man is powerful and effective" (James 5:16). "The LORD is far from the wicked but he hears the prayer of the righteous" (Proverbs 15:29).

> The eyes of the LORD are on the righteous and
> his ears are attentive to their cry; the face of

the LORD is against those who do evil, to cut off the memory of them from the earth. The righteous cry out, and the LORD hears them; he delivers them from all their troubles. The LORD is close to the brokenhearted and saves those who are crushed in spirit. A righteous man may have many troubles, but the LORD delivers him from them all (Psalm 34:15–19).

Notice the requirement for God to be attentive, to hear you, and deliver you from all of your troubles is righteousness. The unrighteous don't have God's ear, nor do they have the benefit of His power to rescue them from trouble. Thus to pray from a state of unrighteousness is to pray ineffectively, and you must diligently avoid this.

Timing is the second condition to consider. Once again, we've all prayed earnestly for something that didn't happen and then began to question God for not answering our prayer, only to find out later that pieces were set in motion from the moment we prayed and merely took time to come together for our prayer to be answered the right way. I've been guilty of this many times. I've prayed diligently for what I thought was the solution and was frustrated when God didn't answer my prayer. Then I felt quite sheepish when God answered my prayer and worked out my problem in an entirely different, far better way, at the perfect time, which was never when I expected. Keep this in mind and be patient. Also praying the same prayer over and over again with more and more passion will not make God move any faster. Trust in Him that He heard you and He will answer your prayer in His timing if it is indeed His will.

God's will is the third condition to consider. God's will always supersedes our own. Thus it is imperative that you pray in accordance with God's will; otherwise, you will be praying ineffectively and wasting your time. The Bible says,

"This is the confidence we have in approaching God: that if we ask anything according to his will, he hears us. And if we know that he hears us—whatever we ask—we know that we have what we asked of him" (1 John 5:14–15). Of course, you have to know God's will if you are to pray according to God's will. This is why studying God's Word and being receptive and listening during prayer is so important.

One of the most common ways people pray ineffectively is in asking God to remove their urge to sin and/or to intervene and prevent them from sinning. Those battling homosexuality like Vicky Beeching pleaded with God to remove their homosexuality, but this is not an effective prayer. Why didn't God comply? Because even if He did remove homosexuality from the individual, that individual's sinful problems would still persist because homosexuality isn't the root of the problem, the sinful nature is. When you recognize that, then you can pray effectively. God will not do anything for you that He's commanded you to do for yourself. You are responsible for your own actions, and as I've said repeatedly, sin is a choice, which means you can choose whether or not you will sin. It is therefore a waste of time to pray for God to stop you from indulging in homosexuality, as though He is going to miraculously put up shields all around you to keep you from sinning. There is wisdom in praying for God to *help* you as you commit to abstaining from sin, but the responsibility still falls on your shoulders. Although righteousness through Christ is a free gift you are still obligated to accept that gift and then maintain that gift through a Christian lifestyle. When you are righteous and seeking God with the right motives, you will not pray ineffectively, and you will be blessed and victorious as a result.

### 3. Don't Succumb to Negative Influences

I'm sure you've heard the saying, "Misery loves company." Well, error loves company too. Immoral people take comfort in surrounding themselves with immoral friends because it makes their lifestyle seem less immoral. However, as soon as someone in that group stands up and says, "This is wrong, I'm not doing this anymore," that causes the others to feel uncomfortable. That declaration of change forces those in error to face reality and consider they also need to change and start doing what's right, but since they aren't ready to change, they don't want anyone around them to change either. I've seen it time and time again in many areas: whether it's a person who decides to stop eating poorly, drinking alcohol, doing drugs, partying, or going to clubs, it appears there's always at least one person who immediately challenges their decision and tries to talk them out of it. They say, "Oh, come on, you're no fun. You're not hurting anyone. You only live once, so you might as well enjoy it." In fact, some people won't rest until the person attempting to change gives up and stays the way they are. It is no different for those fighting to overcome homosexuality.

I recently saw a video documenting the experience of a "lesbian" who decided to give church a try for the first time and came to know Jesus in the process. She explained how through her experience she understood that homosexuality was wrong, and in totally surrendering to Christ she broke up with her girlfriend and told her to move out so that she could focus on living right and pleasing God. While this young lady gained incredible support from her pastors and church family, she immediately experienced great opposition from her friends and people in the "LGBT" community who were angered by her decision to abandon the homosexual lifestyle. People actually responded by saying, "That is so sad. God loves you exactly the way He created you. Just be who you are, don't let anyone else tell you who you're supposed to be, and don't change for anyone." In other words: "God created you to be 'gay', and He loves you, so keep being 'gay.'" Fortunately, for the young lady in the video, she didn't allow this erroneous council to discourage her from following through on her positive decision, and you cannot allow anyone to discourage you in such fashion either. The same cannot be said for countless others who succumb to pressure and poor counsel of their immoral peers. Some of these counselors have unsavory intentions (they know homosexuality is wrong but they don't care), others actually mean well but don't realize in their effort to help, they're actually causing more damage. In the end, those who lean on the council of pro-homosexuals while struggling to overcome homosexuality fail because they ultimately choose to abandon the solution instead of abandoning the problem. What neither the counselor nor the struggler rarely consider is that they will both be held accountable for their actions when they stand before God. The counselor will be judged for leading and encouraging people into sin, and the struggler will be judged for ignoring God's commands and listening to the deceitful counsel of the ungodly. Just as Eve was not absolved of her actions by blaming the serpent in the Garden of Eden, anyone who chooses to continue indulging in homosexuality will not be absolved of their actions by blaming those who encouraged them to do so.

Another way people succumb to negative influences is to be led astray by authors and individuals of notoriety who promote homosexuality. The more the individual struggling with homosexuality accepts false information from what he or she considers credible sources, the faster they fall back into the prison of homosexuality. Again, Vicky Beeching is an example of this. I was fascinated to see that she, along with Pastor Chris, and Matthew Vines all took the exact same approach in convincing themselves that homosexuality is morally acceptable. In their research they committed the *Confirmation Bias* fallacy, which is to reach a conclusion *first,* then ignore everything that conflicts with that conclusion while accepting everything that agrees with that conclusion. Any theologian who supports homosexuality and any book written by a supporter of homosexuality (especially Christian authors) instantly became tools to add credence to their position. This clearly isn't credible scholarship.

As an example of the deception this can cause, Vicky Beeching posted an article on her personal blog titled, "LGBT Theology: What Does the Bible Say?"[46]. The title and article are both wrought with problems. Firstly, the term "LGBT Theology" makes absolutely no sense because *theology* literally means "the study of God." So this translates to "LGBT the study of God." That makes no sense whatsoever, but Vicky strategically attempts to link these two things together in an effort to insist that they are somehow compatible. They aren't. Secondly, and equally as shocking, despite the words "What does the Bible Say," Vicky never actually answered the question by including what the Bible says about homosexuality. Instead, she claimed short blog posts weren't "suited" to the theology on homosexuality (which is ridiculous because people blog about homosexuality all the time) but assured everyone that her new book is the proper venue for such a discussion. She then provided a host of recommended sources: a pair of video clips, both by Matthew Vines, and a list of books that accept and promote homosexuality in the church, and once again Matthew Vines' book was on the list. Oddly enough, the books she selected are among the *exact ones* that Pastor Chris recommended I read. Further, the Bible was not on either of their lists. Be careful, my brothers and sisters. Even if there were a million books written by Christian authors who had multiple PhDs promoting homosexuality, homosexuality would still be sinful. *Appealing to Popularity* and *Appealing to Authority* are also logical fallacies that have absolutely no bearing on what is actually the truth; they do, however, have everything to do with eliciting support to bolster one's own preconceived notions regardless of the truth.

What does this mean for you? The battle of overcoming homosexuality is yours to win or lose. When you stand before

God to give an account for your life you cannot pass the blame on your family your friends or the authors of books that said homosexuality was okay. You are responsible for your decisions and you will be held accountable for those decisions. This means it doesn't matter if the entire world is for you or the entire world is against you, the outcome is still in *your* hands. So keep your guard up from the beginning. Establish up front that failure isn't an option and you will not allow anyone or anything to hinder you from being successful. Encourage yourself. Don't seek out individuals who rationalize homosexuality and follow in their footsteps, seek out individuals who have successfully overcome homosexuality and follow in theirs instead. Find inspiration from godly resources, remain uplifted, and be so determined to be victorious that even if you have to fight all alone, you know you'll still win because you'll never quit, and you'll never fail. This is the attitude and mindset of a victor. Victory can be yours if you desire it so much that you commit to achieving it no matter how hard or how long you have to fight for it.

## 4. Don't Attempt to Change Without Changing

This is what I call kicking the can. The crime here is to start with a good intention: to make a positive and necessary lifestyle change from a practicing "homosexual" to a practicing Christian. Then, due to trepidation or any number of other reasons, the actual change keeps getting delayed, as if the transition is a lengthy process instead of an instantaneous commitment. Let's be clear here: the transition from sinner to Christian is made the instant you truly dedicate your life to God and accept Christ into your heart. After that is when the work starts, and with God's help you have the power to overcome your previous sinful lifestyle. The transition is instantaneous, and yet people like to draw this out as if they have to work up to becoming a Christian first, and then once they're good enough, then they'll fully commit to Christianity and leave their sinful lifestyle behind for good. This never works because you can never be good enough to become a Christian. Salvation is a free gift from God that is not earned but accepted. Moreover, you cannot overcome your sinful nature without being completely dedicated to God.

Anyone who has consistently challenged an addict to change is well aware of the litany of excuses they use to appease you without actually changing. They present strategies to overcome their addiction, which are overly complex, systematic, and take a significant amount of time to actually complete. This is done on purpose so that any time a new challenge comes, the addict can simply say, "I'm working on it," or "I'm making progress." This behavior is destructive and a precursor to failure because addictions are increasingly dangerous, and sin is the most dangerous addiction of all. Imagine one of your loved ones is addicted to a sweet tasting poison. You plead with them to change, and they tell you that they will over a period of time. They promise to drink a little less poison every day until the day they don't drink any at all. At first this sounds like progress, until it occurs to you that they are still drinking poison every day! Sin is the same way. It's not something to play around with or wean yourself off because it never remains stagnant within you. The more you sin, the worse it affects you, and the more powerful your sinful nature becomes. Heaven forbid something tragic happens and you die before you're able to finally change and be completely done with your sinful lifestyle. Considering that did happen, what exactly would you say to God? How would you explain the fact that you refused to give up homosexuality and instead kept kicking the can and continued sinning all the way to your death? At that point there is no hope, no solution, no salvation. There is nothing but eternal destruction. Those who kick the can either accept this fact, or they can ignore this sobering reality and continue to procrastinate. "Nothing will happen to me. I'll change one day," they say, but year after year they fail to overcome their sinful lifestyle.

Another argument I've heard is one of avoidance and appeasement: "I'm trying to change." While this sounds noble on the surface, it's an excuse a lot of people use to continue doing what they're not supposed to do. If they convince themselves that it's a work in progress and they convince everyone else of the same, then that takes the pressure off of actually changing. This defeats the whole purpose. You can't *try* to change without actually *changing* anything. This holds true in every area of life. An obese person can imagine being thin and imagine eating healthy and exercising all day long, but until that person actually commits to dieting and exercising, they will not lose any weight. If we need to change, which we all do in some area, we cannot *try* to do it; we must *do* it. So once you determine you need to overcome homosexuality, commit to overcoming homosexuality, and in doing so you'll stop making excuses and leaving room for sin.

Another common excuse people use to avoid changing is by evoking God's forgiveness. Only those who completely misunderstand God's forgiveness fall into this trap and fail miserably as a result. God forgives those who are honest about their sin and commit to doing whatever it takes to not repeat that sin. God does not forgive those who sin and think by saying, "God forgive me," they are washed clean and can repeat this process to their heart's content. Repentance isn't merely about being absolved of sin; it's about changing in order to keep from sinning in the future. So don't try to take advantage of God's forgiveness. You can't love sin and ask God to rescue you from sin. God knows your heart (your thoughts, will, and motives), and so your intentions are no mystery. He is well aware if you're fighting with every ounce of your strength and will stop at nothing to overcome homosexuality, or if you're simply pretending to fight while procrastinating to avoid making the drastic change you know you need to make.

One of my good friends is an "ex-lesbian." When she first began struggling with homosexuality, she continued to fail because she attempted to change without changing anything. She continued going out to "gay bars" and hanging around her girlfriend and other "lesbians" and wondered why she still struggled to overcome homosexuality. It wasn't until she decided to stop kicking the can and stop surrounding herself with homosexuality that she was able to overcome it. Now she too is happily married and is currently raising her beautiful child with her husband. Remember it all starts in the mind. Purity in mind results in purity in actions. However, one cannot mentally assent to a lifestyle change and expect that change to actually manifest. One cannot carry the mentality of a sinner into the lifestyle of a Christian and expect to experience a difference. You will not see change until you fully commit to changing; then that change will manifest in your thoughts, speech, and actions. Once that change has taken place, it can be maintained through focus, consistency, and undying persistence.

### 5. Don't Obey Feelings Instead of God

You simply cannot be irrational and successfully overcome homosexuality. Sinful feelings are the product of the sinful nature. Therefore, one cannot possibly obey their sinful feelings, commit sin, and believe God either caused this or condones this. I've addressed irrationality at length, and I've pointed out how leaning to one's feelings, opinions, and interpretations is a dangerous recipe for disaster. The danger is far greater when people base their lifestyle not on the truth of God's Word, but on their own feelings and opinions. The irrational thinking goes as follows:

1. I have these feelings.
2. I've tried everything to rid myself of these feelings.
3. I still have these feelings.

4. Therefore these feelings are good (or even from God), and so I accept these feelings and I'm justified in acting on these feelings.

The irrationality of such reasoning is obvious. Failure to eliminate feelings in no way indicates that those feelings are good or they come from God. Millions of people surrender their lives to their feelings, instead of surrendering their lives to God. If one's feelings conflict with God's Word, then those feelings are sinful and acting on those feelings is sinful. True Christians understand we are obligated to do what is right, to remain faithful to God's Word regardless how we feel and regardless of the circumstances. We do not lean to our own understanding or succumb to our sinful feelings. We trust wholeheartedly in God and are led by the Holy Spirit, which is a sign of those who are saved: "those who are led by the Spirit of God are sons of God. For you did not receive a spirit that makes you a slave again to fear, but you received the Spirit of sonship" (Romans 8:14-15).

Indulging in homosexuality is violating God's Moral Law, so you can't keep defending or rationalizing that behavior any longer. I've often heard it argued: "I can't help how I feel," or, "I can't change the way I feel." The truth is our feelings don't supersede God's commands. Further, this argument is not only invalid here, but in every other area. Can a man say, "I can't help but feel sexually attracted to the babysitter" and use that as a means to justify cheating on his wife and carrying on an adulterous relationship with the babysitter? Absolutely not. Can a man who has sexual feelings toward his sister rationalize indulging in incest? Absolutely not. Once again sin is not permitted or condemned based on how you *feel*. Feelings lead us astray. God doesn't. It's not about what you think, or what you like, or what you want. It's all about God and His Word. So regardless of how you feel, you are still obligated to be obedient.

In addition, feelings aren't consistent or immutable. This means we can absolutely change our feelings. We've all done it countless times in our lives in various areas. Even the most powerful feelings can be tamed and changed over time. Some of the most powerful feelings I've had toward females in my past I thought I'd never be rid of. Yet I was wrong in every single case, and now I realize those feelings were so off base I wonder how I ever had them in the first place.

The fear, as I've come to learn, is many "homosexuals" assume if they deny their feelings and impulses toward members of the same sex, they are denying themselves the opportunity to fall in love and find happiness. This is simply untrue because there are plenty of examples of "ex-gays" who are now happily married with children, and there are also "ex-gays" who have chosen to remain celibate and are happy to focus all of their love on God. While many turn up their nose at this idea (which I was once guilty of), the Apostle Paul not only lived a single life of celibacy, fully dedicated to God, but he recommended that lifestyle over marriage. I struggled with this in my own life until I realized not everyone is meant to fall in love and get married. So to sin in order to possibly reach that goal is foolish. Now, after seeking God first and overcoming those powerful urges to have sex, I absolutely love the single life. I love the freedom and stress-free nature of being single. So don't keep practicing a sinful lifestyle and defend it by saying it's the only path to love and happiness because that's not true. Don't cater to sinful feelings; change your sinful feelings and remain faithful to God.

### 6. Don't Give In to Temptation

Once again, Christianity is not something one tries out; Christianity is a lifestyle. In fact, it is the lifestyle that is directly opposed to the sinful lifestyle. Therefore the, "I tried it and it didn't work," mentality fails entirely because "trying" Christianity is something people who are still in love with sin do. You either commit to Christianity or you don't; there is no in between.

Overcoming homosexuality must be approached in the exact same way. One cannot dip their toe in the pool of righteousness and when it starts to feel uncomfortable back away and say, "I tried it and it didn't work." Yet this is exactly what many people do. They shrug their shoulders and say, "I've done everything I can think of: I've gone to church, I've read my Bible, I've tried to find the opposite sex attractive, I've even prayed countless times, but nothing has changed, so how can God possibly condemn me for being the way I am if He won't help me?" At this point many people either give in to temptation and abandon God to indulge in homosexuality, or they reason that God didn't answer their prayer because it is not His will that they be a "heterosexual," and so they return to homosexuality. Both of these are grave mistakes that result in failure. In order to overcome any sinful lifestyle, giving in to temptation is simply not an option. We cannot afford to lean to our own understanding and assume there is only one option available to us when we don't yet experience the victory we seek. It is faulty reasoning to say, "Well, I've struggled for years and have seen no change, so the only option available is to give in and be a 'homosexual.'" No. There is another option: to fight for as long as it takes, refusing to ever give in to temptation until you overcome homosexuality altogether. This is the option "ex-gays" and everyone on the mission to remain sexually pure have chosen. This is the option you must choose regardless of your level of temptation.

Some people blame temptation on God, others blame temptation on the devil, and they use these as excuses to fall back into sin. The fact is we cannot blame our sinfulness on the temptation we face because regardless of how tempted we might be, we still have the option to say "No, I'm not going to do it," and refuse to sin. Nobody forces us to do anything. We choose what we do and what we don't do. Moreover, the book of James reveals to us where temptation comes from and what it leads to.

> When tempted, no one should say, "God is tempting me." For God cannot be tempted by evil, nor does he tempt anyone; but each one is tempted when, by his own evil desire, he is dragged away and enticed. Then, after desire has conceived, it gives birth to sin; and sin, when it is full-grown, gives birth to death (James 1:13–15).

You are the source of your own temptation. Remember, you cannot try to stop entertaining sinful thoughts while surrounding yourself with sinful things and feeding yourself on sinfulness. Otherwise, your temptation will slowly mount until you are powerless to resist it, and then you'll wind up sinning and wonder why you couldn't stop yourself. Preventing this requires you clean house. "Let us purify ourselves from everything that contaminates body and spirit, perfecting holiness out of reverence for God" (2 Corinthians 7:1). Rid yourself of everything in your possession that deals with homosexuality: sex toys, pornography, pictures on your phone, computer, and tablets, premium cable, magazine subscriptions, etc. Shut the door on any and every sexual thing that you've used to feed yourself. Don't just put these things in a box and put them in your closet. Throw them away, cancel them, and delete them. Commit to being celibate immediately by determining you will no longer engage in sexual activity or anything that leads to sexual activity: masturbation, kissing, touching, or flirtation. You must also cut every individual out of your life who stands in the way of your freedom from homosexuality, regardless if it's your partner, your best friend, your pastor, or even a family member. In order to make this drastic change, drastic steps must be taken.

So what happens after you commit to being celibate, you separate yourself from everything that might entice you to return to homosexuality and then you start to feel those old sexual urges? What happens when that temptation begins to mount? First of all, in these cases most people allow those sexual urges to live in their minds and they begin to entertain thoughts about what they feel like doing, what they wish they could do, what they used to do etc. This is a critical mistake! When the temptation mounts the first thing to do is to keep your thoughts pure and reestablish your commitment to not act on any sexual urges. Secondly you have to break this mentality that every sexual urge must be satisfied instead of resisted. You simply cannot continue to live your life based on sexual urges; master your flesh and overcome your flesh so you can be pure and godly despite any and every sexual urge. The Bible says:

> But among you there must not be even a hint of sexual immorality, or any kind of impurity, or of greed, because these are improper for God's holy people. For of this you can be sure: No immoral, impure or greedy person—such a man is an idolater—has any inheritance in the kingdom of Christ and of God (Ephesians 5:3, 5).

This leaves no room for a gray area. "Not even a hint" means if you have to pause to question it, you shouldn't be doing it. So eliminate your sinful desires that are the precursor to temptation. Then, whatever you do, no matter how powerful your urges are, never give in to temptation because it only leads right back to enslavement by the sinful nature followed by death and eternal destruction. Trust me, I know this isn't easy, but I too have had to master temptation and determine no matter what the circumstances are, no matter how I feel or how powerful my urges are, I will not sin. I absolutely refuse to sin. Until you can reach this place and overcome temptation every single time, then you will fail in overcoming homosexuality.

## 7. Don't Make Negative Confessions

Words are more significant than we realize. Words have the power to change reality: they affect us and the world around us. This is how God operates, this is how Jesus Christ operated, this is how the disciples operated, and this is how we must operate. My dad put it this way, "The man who says, 'I can,' and the man who says, 'I can't' are both right." You have what you say, and you are what you say. Romans 10:10 establishes this pattern for us to follow. "For it is with your heart that you believe and are justified, and it is with your mouth that you confess and are saved." The combination of belief and confession in agreement with God's Word is a powerful force that incites change. We find examples of this principle time and time again in Scripture, and it is something that you must master. This means you have to believe in the solution so much that you stop speaking the problem and start speaking the solution. This applies to your ability to change and abandon homosexuality with the power of Christ. Those who believe in their hearts and say, "I not only *can* overcome homosexuality, I *will* overcome homosexuality," are correct. Just as those who lack faith and continue to doubt and say, "I want to overcome homosexuality but I don't think I can," are also correct. So make positive confessions instead of negative ones. Agree with God's Word, and stand on His Word with confidence even when you don't feel it or feel like doing it. This is the secret to speaking change into your life. In combination with your own positive confessions the following Scriptures are excellent examples to speak out loud and stand on:

- "I can do all things through Christ who strengthens me" (Philippians 4:13).

- "I will always obey your law, for ever and ever. I will walk about in freedom, for I have sought out your precepts" (Psalm 119:44–45).
- "I have kept my feet from every evil path so that I might obey your word. I have not departed from your laws, for you yourself have taught me" (Psalm 119:101–102).
- "I made a covenant with my eyes not to look lustfully at a girl [or a guy]" (Job 31:1).
- "I will walk in my house with a blameless heart. I will set before my eyes no vile thing. The deeds of faithless men I hate; they will not cling to me. Men of perverse heart shall be far from me; I will have nothing to do with evil" (Psalm 101:2–4).
- "In all these things we are more than conquerors through him who loved us" (Romans 8:37).
- "For God has not given us a spirit of fear, but of power and of love and of a sound mind" (2 Timothy 1:7).
- "If God is for us, who can be against us?" (Romans 8:31).
- "All things work together for good to those who love God" (Romans 8:28).
- "Commit to the Lord whatever you do, and your plans will succeed" (Proverbs 16:3).
- "Consider it pure joy, my brothers, whenever you face trials of many kinds, because you know that the testing of your faith develops perseverance. Perseverance must finish its work so that you may be mature and complete, not lacking anything" (James 1:2–4).
- "Blessed is the man who perseveres under trial, because when he has stood the test, he will receive the crown of life that God has promised to those who love him" (James 1:12).

- "Let us not become weary in doing good, for at the proper time we will reap a harvest if we do not give up" (Galatians 6:9).

# Summary

I've presented a list of fourteen steps that will result in overcoming homosexuality. It is imperative to keep in mind this list is not a collection of good ideas or recommendations to consider. This list doubles as the mandatory steps necessary for overcoming homosexuality as well as instructions for living a Christian lifestyle. Not a single step can be skipped. Also, don't go through each step as though it's a checklist you have to work your way through and think once you check off step fourteen, your work is done. These are principles to adopt for life; these are practices to maintain indefinitely. If you're about to embark on this journey of overcoming homosexuality, then you have made a wise decision. Now that you've carefully examined each step, prepare yourself for what is to come. The process will not be easy; so don't be surprised when things get difficult. Expect difficulty, but also expect to successfully overcome those difficulties because now you are fully equipped for success. Victory is not something that will be handed to you. It's something you have to fight to acquire and then fight to keep. It is through this relentless fighting that you will find success, freedom, joy, peace, and victory that only God can provide and only God's children can enjoy.

# 12

## Going Forward

We've covered a considerable amount of material in analyzing homosexuality and the impact it has on individuals, children, families, and society as a whole. We've also covered the spiritual impact of homosexuality and the eternal consequences that inevitably follow. What comes next will vary depending on whether you are personally struggling with homosexuality, you fall into the category of an advocate, or you fall into the category of a sympathetic Christian.

## To those Struggling with Homosexuality

The first thing to realize is if you find yourself struggling with homosexuality, then that is a good sign. You cannot be at peace while indulging in sin because God is letting you know that there is something within you that needs to be fixed. There is nothing God wants more than to have a relationship with you, so He's going to help you as much as you allow Him to. He will not force His will on you; it is up to you to repent of your sins and accept the free gift of salvation through Jesus Christ. Embracing sin is to reject Christ, and we must embrace Christ in order to embrace eternal life. Otherwise, embracing sin is embracing eternal destruction. Just as I fight every day to stay pure and to keep myself from sinning sexually and in every area, fight every day to stay pure and keep from sinning sexually and in every other area as well. Don't give in to your sinful nature, not even a little bit, not even for a second. There is hope and victory in Christ. If it is possible to overcome homosexuality (which has been proven and can be seen in lives of countless people), then it is possible for you. Maintain a pure mind. The pattern of homosexuality is the recognition of same-sex attraction, followed by erotic same-sex thoughts, followed by erotic same-sex actions. To break this pattern you have to abstain from "homosexual" actions, devote your mind to Godly thoughts instead of "homosexual" thoughts, and offer God a pure heart to work on in dealing with the same-sex attraction. When you do everything you can do, and *keep* your faith in God, He will do His part and rescue you from your sinful struggle. I offer you my full support as your brother in Christ. I love you and I have faith that you can overcome homosexuality and experience freedom in Christ Jesus.

## To Advocates

I know many people who are absolutely fascinated by the "LGBT" community. They are obsessed with the culture and think "homosexuals" are hilarious, colorful, and entertaining, which prompts them to be staunch supporters of homosexuality, regardless of the fact that it is sinful. Perhaps you can relate to this. Regardless of the reasons, until this point you have been a proponent of homosexuality. Having such a passion and love for "homosexuals" is an awesome thing, but direct that to them in the right way. Invest in helping and saving them by leading them to Christ instead of defending their behavior in an effort to protect their feelings. Which is a more important goal: causing them to feel accepted and equal to everyone here on earth, or showing them how to please God and secure their place in heaven? It's pointless to do the former and sacrifice the latter. Of course, it is noble and commendable to desire to help "homosexuals," but help them the right way. Some of you, in your effort to help "homosexuals" have now seen how you've actually taken a dangerous position that directly opposes God while encouraging others to do the same. Hopefully now you will change your heart and not be focused on defending homosexuality, but on guiding and rescuing those who identify as "homosexuals."

Other advocates may still remain unconvinced homosexuality is sinful or immoral, and their irrational thoughts (their feelings and opinions) overpower their rational thoughts and dismiss the logical conclusions we've reached altogether. This is a part of the struggle for those who are incredibly passionate about promoting homosexuality because they feel it is right. My challenge to those in this position is to remain focused on the truth. Isaiah 5:19–20 says, "Woe to those who call evil good and good evil, who put darkness for light and light for darkness, who put bitterness for sweet and sweet for bitter. Woe to those who are wise in their own eyes and clever in their own sight." So don't lean to your own understanding and give in to irrationality because of your feelings on homosexuality. Work on remaining rational and logical despite your feelings and opinions. As we've seen, opinions and feelings are unreliable because they fluctuate, but the truth sets us on the right path because it is consistent. So ask God to help you to not only understand these principles concerning homosexuality but to embrace them instead of resisting and rejecting them. Ask God to touch your heart *and* your mind so you do not find yourself embracing and defending sinfulness instead of godliness. Then you will be in the best position to help your "homosexual" loved ones the right way by not being an advocate of homosexuality, but by being a loving Christian who is passionate about saving people from homosexuality. Also keep your own eternity in mind. Surely you don't want to find yourself fighting in favor of sinfulness here on earth, which is rejecting God, and expect Him to accept you once you face eternity. Accept God, agree with God, and obey Him from this moment forward. Accept God on earth, and He will accept you in Heaven.

## To Sympathetic Christians

As previously stated, some Christians have simply opted to remain silent regarding homosexuality in order to avoid any arguments or offending anyone. I trust now you can see why that is not an option. Our goal as Christians is not to enable "homosexuals" or to appease homosexuality by remaining silent, but to agree with God and save those struggling with homosexuality in a loving and non-offensive way. This does not mean we need to constantly quote Scriptures, present logical arguments, or list the consequences of homosexuality to prove homosexuality is sinful. At the very least we should constantly be praying for them, and simply remember to be led by the Holy Spirit to say what God wants us to say when He wants us to say it. Proverbs 11:30 says, "he who wins souls is wise." The wise are those who trust in God and are willing to be used by Him. Just as we are sympathetic to sinners in any other area and will do whatever we can to help them and save them, we cannot afford to treat practicing "homosexuals" any differently. We must be willing to be used by God as led by the Holy Spirit to help anyone who struggles with homosexuality and to help advocates understand the truth about homosexuality so they can stop defending and promoting it. Prior to reading this book you may have had no idea how to broach the subject or what to say to help someone struggling with this area, but hopefully you are now fully equipped to be used by God to make tremendous changes in people's lives.

# Conclusion

The topic of homosexuality is commonly misunderstood and mishandled and that needs to change. We need to be logical and rational and approach the topic of homosexuality from the most important perspective, which is morality. My prayer is anyone who has struggled with the topic of homosexuality, wrestled with unanswered questions, and/or avoided the issue is now well informed and fully equipped to tackle this issue head on in a loving and respectful manner. For those who are battling homosexuality, my prayer is you now have everything you need to overcome homosexuality and to help others do so as well. I'll leave you with just a few bullet points to sum up all that we've learned:

- Only a perfect moral agent can establish a universal Moral Law, and none of us are perfect moral agents.
- Morality is objective, and when it comes to objectivity opinions are irrelevant.
- True Christians honor God in public *and* in the privacy of their own homes.
- Upon hearing the truth, one can either accept it or reject it, but rejecting the truth has absolutely no effect on the truth.

- If the truth offends you, then you are living outside the truth.
- Attraction does not justify the indulgence in the object of that attraction.
- Immoral conduct resulting from a predisposition does not become moral conduct as a result; nor can immoral conduct be rationalized based on that predisposition.
- Either Christ is your Lord and you fully obey his word, or He isn't and you don't.
- Disliking, misunderstanding, and/or disagreeing with God's commands don't alter His commands or excuse us from following them.
- Society and popular opinion don't override God's commands.
- Those who try to adjust God's Word to suit their sinfulness instead of acknowledging and purging their sinfulness to obey God's Word will suffer terrible consequences.
- One can either love God and reject sin or love sin and reject God. The two are mutually exclusive and the consequences of each choice are abundantly clear in Scripture.
- God's love is not predicated on one's moral status, nor does God's love excuse one's immoral status.
- God loves us unconditionally, and until we love Him unconditionally in return, we will never be free from sin.
- Sin is a choice, which means we can all choose to not practice sin. We may not be able to choose the cards we're dealt in life, but we can certainly choose how we play those cards.
- We are judged not by how we were born, but by how we live. If we were judged by how we were born, we would all go to hell.

- In response to homosexuality, our primary goal as Christians is to save "homosexuals" in a loving, non-offensive way.
- True love doesn't justify sin, nor does it lead to sin. If the result of your "love" is sin, then it's not love; it's lust.
- Love is not ignoring or enabling our neighbors' sinfulness; love is helping our neighbors abstain from sinfulness.
- God is *always* right. If you disagree with God, then you're wrong.
- There are no circumstances that excuse sinful behavior. We are all obligated to be good people and do what is right at all times regardless of the circumstances.
- The notion that all sexual urges must be satisfied one way or another is false. Sexual urges can and must be resisted if satisfying those sexual urges results in sin.
- "Ex-gays" not only exist, they outnumber "gays."
- It is possible to overcome homosexuality, and if it is possible, then it is possible for you.

# REFERENCES

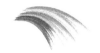

1. Ravi K Zacharias, The End of Reason : A Response to the New Atheists, (Grand Rapids, Mich. : Zondervan, 2008), p. 41.
2. http://barbwire.com/2014/06/02/needs-featured-image-barbwire-author-21-questions-tolerance-crowd/
3. http://www.gallup.com/poll/183383/americans-greatly-overestimate-percent-gay-lesbian.aspx?utm_source=Social%20Issues&utm_medium=newsfeed&utm_campaign=tiles
4. http://youtu.be/8TJxnYgP6D8
5. http://www.queerty.com/can-we-please-just-start-admitting-that-we-do-actually-want-to-indoctrinate-kids-20110512
6. http://fellowshipoftheminds.com/tag/daniel-villarreal/
7. http://ne.general.narkive.com/4hgRrare/making-schools-safe-means-refashioning-values-in-massachusetts
8. http://m.christianpost.com/news/why-i-take-controversial-stands-and-debate-our-cultural-decline—131390/
9. http://www.massresistance.org/docs/marriage/effects_of_ssm_2012/index.html.
10. http://www.washingtonpost.com/opinions/im-gay-i-want-my-kid-to-be-gay-too/2015/02/19/eba697c2-b847–11e4-aa05–1ce812b3fdd2_story.html.

11. Thomas E. Schmidt, *Straight and Narrow?* (Downer's Grove, IL.: InterVarsity Press, 1995), chapter 6, 108.
12. D. McWhirter and A. Mattison, "The Male Couple: How Relationships Develop" (Englewood Cliffs, Prentice-Hall, 1984).
13. Paul Van de Ven et al., "A Comparative Demographic and Sexual Profile of Older Homosexually Active Men," *Journal of Sex Research* 34 (1997): 354."
14. http://www.cnn.com/2014/11/23/politics/terry-bean-sex-abuse-charges/.
15. http://www.smh.com.au/national/named-the-australian-paedophile-jailed-for-40-years-20130630-2p5da.html.
16. http://www.abc.net.au/news/2014–03–10/boy-with-henna-tattoo-network-exposed/5310812.
17. http://nambla.org/welcome.html.
18. www.huffingtonpost.co.uk/2014/07/11/australian-judge-garry-neilson-suspended-incest-abortion-remarks_n_5577090.html.
19. http://nypost.com/2014/04/23/married-lesbian-threesome-expecting-first-child/.
20. http://www.charismanews.com/opinion/in-the-line-of-fire/48454-if-love-is-love-why-not-three-men-marrying.
21. http://nymag.com/scienceofus/2015/01/what-its-like-to-date-your-dad.html.
22. http://www.hollanddavis.com/?p=3647.
23. http://www.ldolphin.org/lesbian.html.
24. http://barbwire.com/2015/02/16/change-therapy-scientific-testimony-data-gay-activists-dont-tell/.
25. http://www.amazon.com/The-Queen-James-Bible/dp/0615724531.
26. Richard Dawkins, *River Out of Eden* (New York: Basic Books, 1996), p.133.
27. http://www.skeptical-science.com/essays/science-religion-richard-dawkins/.
28. http://www.cdc.gov/msmhealth/STD.htm.

29. William Lane Craig, *Hard Questions, Real Answers* (Wheaton, IL: Crossway Books, 2003), p. 141.

30. Lettie L. Lockhart et al., "Letting out the Secret: Violence in Lesbian Relationships," *Journal of Interpersonal Violence* 9 (December 1994): 469–492.

31. Gwat Yong Lie and Sabrina Gentlewarrier, "Intimate Violence in Lesbian Relationships: Discussion of Survey Findings and Practice Implications," *Journal of Social Service Research* 15 (1991): 41–59.

32. D. and P. Letellier, *Men Who Beat the Men Who Love Them: Battered Gay Men and Domestic Violence* (New York: Haworth Press, 1991), p. 14.

33. http://www.catholiceducation.org/en/science/faith-and-science/can-immunology-corroborate-the-two-in-one-flesh-image-in-genesis.html.

34. http://www.cancer.org/healthy/find-cancerearly/womenshealth/cancer-facts-for-lesbians-and-bisexual-women.

35. https://www.youtube.com/watch?v=ezQjNJUSraY.

36. http://illinoisfamily.org/homosexuality/"homosexual"-activist-admits-true-purpose-of-battle-is-to-destroy-marriage//

37. http://americansfortruth.com/issues/glbtq-quotes/religious-leaders//

38. http://www.thepublicdiscourse.com/2015/02/14370/.

39. http://www.aleteia.org/en/society/article/351-studies-from-13-nations-prove-benefits-of-households-with-a-dad-a-mom-and-their-kids-5798145510342656.

40. http://thefederalist.com/2015/03/17/dear-gay-community-your-kids-are-hurting/#.VQjagOG-RW5.facebook.

41. http://www.cnsnews.com/news/article/lauretta-brown/adults-raised-gay-couples-speak-out-against-gay-marriage-federal-court#.VQw-Hq7wXUI.facebook.

42. https://www.youtube.com/watch?v=5GivMLlmeAU

43. http://www.independent.co.uk/news/people/news/vicky-beeching-star-of-the-christian-rock-scene-im-gay-god-loves-me-just-the-way-i-am-9667566.html.
44. https://www.youtube.com/watch?v=uQ-GA-n4JyOY&list=FLsPx5w7mD8VSmdtjycyhE2g.
45. http://americansfortruth.com/2007/10/11/ex-lesbian-charlene-cothran-tells-aftah-banquet-that-born-gay-claim-is-vicious-lie/.
46. http://vickybeeching.com/blog/LGBT-theology-2/.

CPSIA information can be obtained
at www.ICGtesting.com
Printed in the USA
BVHW040320050222
627964BV00005B/106

9 781498 443166